Psychology Revivals

Administrative Psychiatry

First published in 1937, *Administrative Psychiatry* was the first book to present theory and practice in a hospital for psychiatric patients. Every detail of the organization and direction of a psychiatric hospital is described in this volume. Everything advocated in this volume had passed the test of actual trial, the principles set forth having been in continuous operation over a period of years before the book was written. A pioneering text at the time, today it can be read in its historical context.

This book is a re-issue originally published in 1937. The language used and views portrayed are a reflection of its era and no offence is meant by the Publishers to any reader by this re-publication.

Administrative Psychiatry

William A. Bryan

Routledge
Taylor & Francis Group
LONDON AND NEW YORK

First published in 1937
by George Allen & Unwin

This edition first published in 2025 by Routledge
4 Park Square, Milton Park, Abingdon, Oxon, OX14 4RN

and by Routledge
605 Third Avenue, New York, NY 10017

Routledge is an imprint of the Taylor & Francis Group, an informa business

Publisher's Note
The publisher has gone to great lengths to ensure the quality of this reprint but points out that some imperfections in the original copies may be apparent.

Disclaimer
The publisher has made every effort to trace copyright holders and welcomes correspondence from those they have been unable to contact.

A Library of Congress record exists under LCCN: 37027130

ISBN: 978-1-032-93669-7 (hbk)
ISBN: 978-1-003-56728-8 (ebk)
ISBN: 978-1-032-93704-5 (pbk)

Book DOI 10.4324/9781003567288

ADMINISTRATIVE PSYCHIATRY

By

WILLIAM A. BRYAN, M.D.
Superintendent Worcester State Hospital
WORCESTER, MASS.

70 Fifth Avenue, New York

FIRST EDITION

This volume is dedicated to my wife,

FLOY GILBERT BRYAN,

who passed many evenings listening to the clack of a typewriter and sustaining and encouraging me in an unfamiliar and laborious task. Her share in the project is no small one, and this acknowledgment is a small part of the debt I owe for her patience and understanding.

INTRODUCTION

The reasons why men write books which embody their own experiences are not always clear, even to the authors. Presumably they have the urge to pass along the information they have acquired in order that others may profit. But the experience of one individual may be of little value to another because of differences in conditions and personalities. Undoubtedly a writer gets a considerable amount of ego satisfaction from seeing his brain-child go forth to spread the gospel of his own theories and beliefs.

To one who has spent a considerable number of years guiding the organization of a mental hospital through the changes that have come in our economic and political life, it becomes increasingly evident that the future of psychiatry and its influence on public health will be built around the hospital. The kind of leadership which the institution gives will depend largely upon the acceptance by administrators of the responsibility for teaching and training younger men who will guide the destinies of the future hospital. The administrator who sees himself as a teacher of others sooner or later becomes paternalistic in his attitude. More and more he gets his compensations in training younger men to accept and carry out greater responsibilities successfully.

If I must give a reason for the presentation of this volume, it is that the above-mentioned feelings have developed and grown stronger with the passing of the years, and the need for a wider audience has appeared. I offer it to the men who have more recently entered the field of psychiatry with the hope that it may be of some value to them in the formulation of their own philosophy of leadership.

There is a distinct scarcity of literature which treats of mental hospital administration. In the psychiatric literature of the world the administrator has been pushed aside by the fascinating speculations of the research worker and the clinical psychiatrist. Yet back of every research project and every clinic there is an executive who builds and maintains the organization without which they cannot survive. He is an essential member of the team. If more administrators were interested in research and more research workers appreciated the importance of administration, the whole field of psychiatry would be benefited immeasurably.

In the general hospital much attention has been given to the theories and principles of organization. A number of splendid books have been written which are available for young men who desire to enter the specialty of administration. More recently an institute has been organized where executives may secure an intensive course in the fundamentals of organization as they relate to the general hospital. But the problems of the psychiatric hospital are so specialized and the type of organization so different that such resources are of little value to those whose specialty is psychiatry. Information relating to psychiatric administration is still passed on by word of mouth, and few textbooks that treat of these problems are available.

The material in this book comes from two sources. It is an elaboration of discussions which have been held weekly over a considerable period of years with the staff of the Worcester State Hospital. To my associates I express deep appreciation for their constant stimulation and for much of the material between these covers. I am also indebted to many writers, particularly those working in the field of industrial psychology. The principles and theories set forth are fundamentally not original. I have attempted to give credit wherever possible. But one is always in danger of unconscious plagiarism, and if I have failed anywhere to acknowledge the source of the material it is not because of a willful desire to use what does not belong to me. I have spent many hours browsing through the literature and many years discussing these matters with my colleagues from other hospitals. To these colleagues I also make grateful acknowledgment.

I may say that practically everything discussed in this book has passed the test of actual trial. It is not the result of abstract, armchair day-dreaming, but the ideas set forth have actually been in operation over a period of years. In the particular setting in which they have been tried and with the personalities involved, all of them have had some degree of success.

I am indebted to Dr. F. H. Sleeper, David Shakow, and Dr. E. M. Jellinek for editorial assistance in the preparation of the manuscript. My thanks are also due to Miss Mary E. Kelly for her secretarial help and advice. To Dr. George L. Banay appreciation is extended for the preparation of the index.

CONTENTS

Chapter 1

DEVELOPMENT OF THE MENTAL HOSPITAL

IF THERE is one thing that stands out clearly in medical history it is the fact that primitive man was completely dominated by his belief in animism. He explained disease and death by the idea that invisible spirits swarmed about him and epidemics of sickness afflicted him because of the wrath of these spirits or deities. The healing art, therefore, could only be carried on through methods by which the malign influence could be propitiated or repelled. Insanity was considered as the possession of the individual by a benevolent or avenging deity.

With this theory, as might be supposed, the treatment of mental disease consisted of religious ceremonies and was in the hands of the priests. In Greece the Asclepiads, the medical priests, were in charge of the temples where sick people were treated. The therapeutic ceremonies have been described in the Hippocratic writings. The temples of Asklepios were scattered far and wide over Greece. They were not devoted exclusively to patients suffering from mental disease but were the forerunners of the modern general hospital. The three that were famous for their cures were at Pergamon, Kos, and Epidauros. The last named was the best known of the three. The excavations which have been carried on at Epidauros have brought to light much information about the plan of the temple and particularly the votive tablets, which are the first medical case records. The site of the temple is very attractive. Evidently this was considered to be of great importance. The temple had one of the finest theaters in all Greece, with a seating capacity of 20,000. In addition there was a stadium with room for 12,000 people. The modern mental hospital invariably has an assembly hall or theater and recreational grounds.

The first building of the sanctuary is an immense square

structure with four courtyards surrounded by small cells. To the left are the gymnasium and baths and close by is the temple proper. The fame of this temple was due to a deep-rooted faith in the healing power of the god. The stelae or stone tablets have been found and translated. They were not only case records but testimonials offered in gratitude for favors received. Each stele contains a number of accounts of cure, but one will serve as an example of all: [1]

"Hermodikes, of Lampsakos, was paralyzed in body. In his sleep he was healed by the God, who ordered him to bring to the temple as large a stone as he could, when he left the Abaton. The man brought the stone which now lies before the Abaton."

Truly the customs of the modern patent medicine vendor are of great antiquity. The patients were received by the physician-priests, who stirred their imagination by telling of the deeds of Asklepios, and the success of the treatment and the remedies employed. After appropriate prayers and sacrifices the patient was further purified by a bath from the mineral spring, with massage, inunction, etc. After the sacrifice of a cock before the image of the god, he was inducted into the special rite known as incubation, or temple sleep. This consisted of lying down to sleep in the sanctuary, where during the night the priest, in the guise of the god, presented himself before the patient to administer medical advice if he should happen to be awake. If he slept, as was usually the case, the advice came in a dream which was afterward interpreted by the priest. He also prescribed catharsis, emesis, blood-letting, or whatever other remedies seemed appropriate. If the treatments were successful, the patient presented a thank-offering to the god. A votive tablet giving the history of the case was suspended in the temple.

There are few records available that show how mental patients were cared for during the Hippocratic era. Whether they were in special establishments and whether restraint or coercion was used cannot be ascertained with accuracy. There is some evidence that would show that asylums did exist.[2] Plutarch speaks of Antiphon, a physician at Corinth, and Herodotus relates the history of a lunatic, Cleomenes, King of Lacedaemon, who, having fallen into a frenzy, with violent agitation, was secured by wooden fetters.

Celsus (*ibid.* p. 11), A.D. 5, wrote at length upon the subject of the treatment of mental disease, and formulated some wise rules as to hygienic and moral management. Unfortunately he advised the use of hunger, chains, and chastisement.

One of the outstanding Greek writers who gives us some indication of the methods of caring for mental patients is Coelius Aurelianus (*ibid.* p. 13), A.D. 195. His accounts of the treatment of insanity are the most complete of any of the writers of this period. He was an advocate of a non-restraint regime. In discussing the treatment then in vogue he says, speaking of physicians:

"They seem rather to lose their own reason than to be disposed to cure their patients when they liken them to wild beasts who must be tamed by the deprivation of food and the torments of thirst. Misled, doubtless, by the same error, they advise the inhuman use of chains, not considering how their members may be lacerated or broken and how much better it is to control by the hands of men than by the often useless weight of iron. They go so far as to counsel bodily violence and blows, as if to compel the return of reason by such provocations, a deplorable method of treatment that can only aggravate the patients' condition, injure them physically, and offer to them the miserable remembrance of their suffering whenever they recover the use of their reason."

He has the following to say about the management of difficult and disturbed patients (*ibid.* p. 15):

"If the sight of other persons irritates them and only in very rare cases, restraint by tying may be employed, but with the greatest precautions without any unnecessary force and after carefully protecting all the joints and with special care to use only restraining apparatus of a soft and delicate texture, since means of repression employed without judgment increase and may even give rise to furor instead of repressing it." These rules could hardly be improved upon even in the present.

Throughout the Middle Ages there was little provision made for mental patients. They were allowed to roam about at will or were confined to prisons, almshouses, and a few asylums, which were actually little better than the jails. The first European mental asylum was Bethlehem Hospital, or Bedlam, as it has always been called. The word has been used generically for all "lunatic asylums." It was founded by Simon Fitz Mary in 1247. Fitz Mary was sheriff of London, and he established the institution as a priory for the brothers and sisters of the order of the Star of Bethlehem. Its actual beginning as a hospital is not known. It is certain that mental patients were confined there in 1403. In 1547 the institution was turned over to the City of London by Henry VIII for the care of lunatics. It became the most infamous place in Europe and was noted for the brutal treatment of patients.

The first medical superintendent of Bethlehem Hospital was John Arundell. He was the chaplain and confessor of Henry VI, but he was also a doctor of medicine and the king's "first physician," and was appointed to the post because of his services to the king. He later became Bishop of Chichester. For a detailed history of this celebrated institution the reader is referred to the exhaustive historical research by Edward Geoffrey O'Donoghue,[3] *The Story of Bethlehem Hospital.* The institution has been in existence continuously since its beginning.

Another celebrated hospital where mental patients were cared for is the Hotel Dieu, in Paris. In 1660 two wards were set aside for insane patients. One, St. Louis, was reserved for men. It contained ten beds for four patients each and two small beds. The St. Martin ward was reserved for females, and contained six large and six small beds. Several beds were set aside for cases of hydrophobia. Treatment of this condition consisted of douches, cold baths, and phlebotomy.

This is probably the first instance of a psychiatric department in a general hospital. Patients were admitted, and if they did not recover in a few weeks they were considered incurable and distributed to the Petites Maisons, the Salpêtrière, or the Bicêtre. There, loaded with chains and collars of iron, with only rags to cover them and rotten straw to lie on, and ill nourished, they dragged out a miserable existence until death relieved their suffering. The public was admitted on holidays on payment of a fee, and visitors were permitted to tease them through the bars of the cages, as they would wild animals.

This was the situation when Philip Pinel became physician to the insane at the Bicêtre in 1793. The conditions that he found were indescribable. The outstanding fact in the life of this great administrator is that he disregarded the pressing problems of administration and sanitation for the more important task of treating the patients. It is significant that when he took over the direction of the Salpêtrière and repeated his experience at the Bicêtre he insisted upon the replacement of the entire attendant personnel. He recognized the difficulty of turning individuals from the traditional attitudes and ways of doing things. This is a lesson that many modern administrators have had to learn. Pinel had the same troubles that beset the present-day executive. The Central Bureau was weak and was reluctant to approve such a radical measure. The struggle to accomplish the removal of these brutal attendants therefore lasted a number of years. During Pinel's incumbency at the Bicêtre he fought the politicians of his day. The courage of the mild little scientist was tried to the limit by this interference. He is truly a model for all mental hospital administrators, not alone for his humanitarianism but for his vision and courage to strike out into untrodden fields. It would be unfair not to mention the faithful and loyal Pussin, who was the instrument through which Pinel worked. It was he who actually organized and carried out many of the administrative reforms. Psychiatry owes a great deal to the initiative and persistent will of these men.

Pinel was not merely a reformer but a man of careful scientific observation. His book, *Faite de la Manie,* can be read with profit today. He advocated many administrative procedures which are used in our present mental hospitals.

Another figure that stands out conspicuously in this psychiatric renaissance is William Tuke, who founded the York Retreat in 1796. The background of that institution was the great humanitarianism of the Quakers. The primary motive back of it was benevolence rather than therapy. The Retreat was not under the direction of a physician, but George Jepson, the first director, recognized the necessity for a medical atmosphere. The emphasis was upon "moral treatment," and careful directions were laid down for the government of the patients. Like the modern superintendent, the Quakers recognized both the importance of the attendants and the difficulty of getting individuals with the requisite temperament and understanding of the patients. The personality of the attendant was considered of prime importance. He was urged not to be familiar with his patients, yet to do everything possible to arouse their affection and confidence. He was not to reason with them during moments of stress, nor was he to speak condescendingly to them in lucid intervals. "The patient is really under the influence of a disease, which deprives him of responsibility and frequently leads him into expressions and conduct the most opposite to his character and natural disposition." [4]

The Quakers realized the difficulties of fulfilling these requirements:—"To consider them (the insane) at the same time both as brothers and as mere automata; to applaud all they do right; and pity, without censuring, whatever they do wrong, requires such a habit of philosophical charity, as is certainly difficult to attain" (*ibid.*).

The influence of these reforms crossed the Atlantic, and American psychiatry was born. Many illustrious names figure prominently in the development of mental hospital administration, which came rapidly following the establishment of the institution at Williamsburg, Virginia, in 1773. Rush, Kirkbride, Earl Wyman, and Woodward were pioneers, not only in psychiatry but in the development of the country. No man can study the history of American psychiatry and not feel humble. The innovations that one fondly believes to be one's own are found to have been tried many years ago. It has been pointed out that the ideas expressed in this book are not new. In an article on "Moral Treatment of Insanity," [5] published in the *Journal of Insanity* in 1847, I find that the author advocates a specialization of attendants. He says:

"We are satisfied that an establishment for the insane can be better managed and with equal economy, by having an arrangement by which some attendants devote their time to the ordinary duties and labors of the halls, while others have nothing to do but to accompany the patients and endeavor to amuse and instruct them. The latter having nothing to do with any coercive measures, the patients do not become prejudiced against them and will readily harken to their suggestions." We see here the forerunner of the nurse-attendant relation or even individual psychotherapy of a kind.

Dr. Wyman,[6] first superintendent of the McLean Hospital, gave an address before the Massachusetts Medical Society on, "Mental Philosophy as Connected with Mental Disorders." In this address he said:

"In mental disorders without symptoms of organic disease, a judicious moral management is most successful. It should afford agreeable occupation. It should engage the mind and exercise the body; as in riding, walking, sewing, embroidering, bowling, gardening, mechanic arts; to which may be added reading, writing, conversation, etc., the whole to be performed with *order and regularity*. Even the taking of food, rising in the morning and at stated times, and conforming to stated rules in almost everything, is a most salutary discipline. It requires, however, constant attention and vigilance, with the greatest kindness in the attendants upon a lunatic. Moral treatment is indispensable, even in cases arising from organic disease." This is the principle of habit training, started at that early date. Administrative psychiatry is not of recent origin.

But it remained for a frail little woman of indomitable will and high purpose to give a real impetus to the American mental hospital movement. Dorothea Lynde Dix, that remarkable woman whom Dr. Tuke characterized as a "terrible reformer but gentle lady," was a contemporary of another pioneer to whom the world owes a great debt of gratitude, Florence Nightingale. There are many points of resemblance between them. Both came from cultured backgrounds. Each was inspired by lofty ideals of humanitarianism and religion. Their reforms were built upon a foundation of actual knowledge and experience, and both possessed great leadership and administrative ability.

To Dorothea Lynde Dix belongs the credit of placing the care of the insane in this country and abroad upon a firm foundation of kind and humane treatment. A fitting tribute to her was written by Francis Tiffany: [7]

"In all her rationality, in all her enthusiasm of humanity, in all her glowing faith in the birth of a new epoch in human history, Miss Dix was the incarnation of the sanguine and prophetic spirit of her time."

In the development of American psychiatry there have been certain definite trends of thought and shifts of leadership. The first organized psychiatry in this country was confined solely to the mental hospitals. In the beginning the humanitarian ideal was in the foreground. Society was actuated by motives of sympathy and pity to take some cognizance of the plight of those who were deviates from the standards of the group and to make provision for their care in custodial institutions. Psychiatry was therefore based largely on kindly care, and hospitals were built with the purpose of providing good physical attention and of segregating these individuals from the community. With segregation and under the influence of the grade of excellent physical care provided, a certain degree of improvement occurred in all patients and even recovery in others. Thus the idea of therapy was born. In this first step hospital administration was the important therapeutic weapon. Fortunately the administration of these mental hospitals was entrusted to physicians whose training helped the rapid development of therapy.

Thus we see that in the early days of American psychiatry the mental hospital assumed the leadership. The earliest psychiatric organization was the Association of Medical Superintendents, organized in 1844 and now known as the American Psychiatric Association. However, the influence of new thought, the development of social work in many forms, the inauguration of mental clinics, the mental hygiene movement, all developed outside the hospital and tended to relegate the institution to the background.

That there was some justification for this movement away from the State hospital there can be little doubt. Mental hospitals became isolated units, having little contact with the communities they served and in most cases being objects of fear and suspicion. The difficulty of travel, which made it hard to get together for mutual discussions, and the traditional resistance of the medical profession to new thought tended to complete the isolation. The importance placed by superintendents upon the economic side of hospital administration had its effect in the failure of the State hospital to see the advantage of a more closely-knit relationship with the community and the necessity of changing the type of leadership which it was giving. The sense of economic security which comes with hospital existence contributed in no small measure to the attitude of satisfaction and smugness that eventually grew up. The physician was supreme. He had no competition. Laymen were not interested in the problems of mental disorder.

But the organization of social service, the increasing contributions by psychology, the newer dynamic conceptions of mental disorder, and the advent of mental hygiene had such possibilities of disturbing the orderly routine of the mental hospital and created such wild experimentations that the new situation was met by a partial withdrawal. Hospital administrators in general avoided embroiling themselves in such controversial subjects, insisting that their business was the proper care of patients, and they continued to give this custodial care thoroughly and well.

However, these movements, bringing psychiatry out into the community, went on in spite of considerable passive resistance. For the past three decades the mental hospital has not been in particularly good standing with forward-looking psychiatry. It has not been an outstanding factor in mental hygiene programs, and it has not attracted the outstanding medical and other professional men; in a word, for some years the mental hospital has been standing still. Around its walls surged the turbulent battles of the psychoanalyst and the organicist, the controversies among followers of Freud, the clamor of the psychologist for his place in the scheme. Through it all the mental hospital went peacefully on "caring for its patients." And perhaps it was wise in doing so. However, it can no longer disregard these movements. They are here to stay, and the State hospital will be wise to search them carefully for the good that is in them. This is not the place for a discussion of the theories of psychoanalysis, but it cannot be doubted that it has a place in the armamentarium of the hospital.

There can be little question that the most potent factor in the development of American psychiatry in this country during the last quarter of a century was the establishment of the National Committee for Mental Hygiene. This organization has inaugurated and is carrying out as rapidly as circumstances will permit a most comprehensive program dealing with all general phases of the mental disease problem. Over a long period of years it has continued its efforts for the betterment of institutional facilities for the mentally ill. Through the activities of the Division of Psychiatric Education the psychiatric departments of an appreciable percentage of medical schools have been improved. The Committee has recognized the necessity for highly trained specialists in the various fields of psychiatry and has provided fellowships which may provide a nucleus for later leadership in this specialty. Through its contacts with great philanthropic organizations, money has been forthcoming for research activities. The Committee has raised large amounts for public education, preventive work, the establishment of child guidance and mental hygiene clinics, and has succeeded in definitely influencing public opinion in its attitude towards the entire problem of mental disease. The relationship of psychiatry and the law has received attention. It has been interested in and contributed to the integration of mental health principles into the practices of social work, nursing, public health administration, education, industry, and government. The Committee conducts mental hygiene and psychiatric institutional surveys and studies.

The preceding list by no means covers all the activities of the National Committee for Mental Hygiene. For a full understanding of the contributions of this organization one should read the articles, "Twenty Years of Mental Hygiene," by George K. Pratt [8] and "Twenty-five Years of Work," by A. H. Ruggles.[9]

What is the place of the hospital in the scheme? The State hospital system of this country is again in a position to assume that leadership of American psychiatry which it formerly had. But that leadership must be constructive, it must be broad and far-sighted. The hospital is the one stable factor. Clinics come and clinics go, organizations for the correction of this and that difficulty come into existence, flourish and fade, but the mental hospital goes on. It can be a tower of strength in the psychiatric world if it will turn its attention to a more active psychiatric leadership, but this leadership will never be accepted if the attitude of disinterestedness in new thought is to continue. Should we not analyze the entire situation with a critical attitude, check up our own shortcomings, and embark upon the future with new perspectives, new charts, and new sailing orders?

Chapter 2

STATE AND HOSPITAL ORGANIZATION

GOVERNMENTAL control of psychiatric hospitals probably grew out of the principle of English common law which placed upon the Crown the duty of "caring for those who cannot take care of themselves." An act passed in the reign of Edward I conferred upon the King the responsibility for the care of idiots and lunatics. The obligation of the ruler was more definitely fixed by the *Statute de Prerogativa Regis* which was passed during the reign of Edward II (A.D. 1342). Today in this country 95 per cent of the patients hospitalized because of mental disease are under the jurisdiction of the several states.

During the past twenty-five years State hospitals have increased more than twofold both in number and in bed capacity. In 1934 the mental institutions of the United States had a bed capacity of 513,845. There was an average of 488,481 inmates for the same year.[10] Since the World War the Federal Government has assumed almost entirely the responsibility for veterans afflicted with mental disease. It is doubtful if many people realize the tremendous contribution the Federal Government has made to the problems of psychiatry. The Veterans' Bureau cares for some 15,000 nervous and mental cases. The Department of the Interior has under its control St. Elizabeth's Hospital with a resident population of 5,000 patients. An excellent article by Walter Treadway,[11] Chief of the Division of Mental Hygiene, U. S. Public Health Service, on "Federal Activities in the Care of the Mentally Ill," brings to our attention some of these governmental agencies. He says, "Of the ten executive departments of the government, eight have functions that are directly and intimately concerned with the problem of mental disease. Only the Post Office Department and the Department of Agriculture have no executive functions concerned with the subject of mental illness."

In August, 1925 the Public Health Service inaugurated a system of examination of prospective immigrants in their native countries. By January, 1931, the system was operating in sixteen foreign countries. In the fiscal year 1928-29 seven out of each thousand examined were excluded because of mental disorder.

In 1929 Congress authorized the establishment of two institutions for the confinement and treatment of persons who are addicted to the use of habit-forming narcotic drugs and who have committed offenses against the United States. The Public Health Service administers these organizations. The service also controls the psychiatric department of the Federal Prisons and is charged with making studies and investigations of causes, prevalence, and means for prevention of nervous and mental diseases. This is a research function that is logically vested in the Federal Government.

It is hardly necessary to comment on the contribution of the Department of Commerce through its Bureau of the Census and Vital Statistics. Since 1926 an annual census has been published, which has served to call attention to the problem in no uncertain way. Psychiatry is the outstanding example of "state medicine" and, as Hamilton [12] points out, organized medicine does not object to governmental agencies handling the problem.

The administration of the institutions housing this great number of patients is an important function of state government. Hospital plants represent an investment of millions of dollars and require millions annually for maintenance and upkeep. The amount needed for personnel and hospital supplies is staggering. If efficient administrative machinery for control is not set up, the inevitable result is waste of public funds and exploitation of the patient. There has been a tendency in many states to place an emphasis on certain material aspects of the problem and to relegate to the background more important considerations which directly affect the treatment of the patients. For instance, a great deal of importance is attached to farm activity and production. There can be no question that farming processes are important from the standpoint of economy, and when utilized properly they are of the greatest value as a therapeutic agent. But to stress the breeding of blue ribbon cattle or the production of prize-winning vegetables and sacrifice medical supplies and equipment is a short-sighted policy.

The custom of judging the administration of hospitals exclusively on the basis of per capita cost is a vicious practice. They can be operated at such low cost that the essential purpose for which they are built is defeated. Excessively low per capita costs are invariably gained by sacrificing many things that would contribute to the recovery of patients. They are accompanied by poor service, which is expensive at any price. Low costs are misleading when they are gained by a refusal to make expenditures needed to protect the investment. When states economize by deferring maintenance charges, they build up a liability which must eventually be met.

The expenditures for the maintenance of our mental hospitals are, in large part, a total loss to the taxpayers of the state, except that they prevent the greater social and economic loss which would result from the failure to provide such care. This loss can be reduced by a strenuous and systematic effort on the part of each state to decrease the demand for increased accommodations through preventive measures applied on a large scale. Such results can only be attained through organization methods and points of view. There are two distinct policies open to the State in dealing with these problems. One offers immediate savings in the cost of maintenance of patients but with the certainty of a continued increase in their number, increased expenditures for additional facilities, and increased demands for the maintenance and operation of the institutions. The other policy offers no immediate saving in unit cost of operation and maintenance but a strong probability that patient population will be decreased and eventually lower costs to a point which could never be achieved by the adoption of the first. A policy of parsimony means limiting the work of the hospital to a purely custodial type of care until death relieves the State of its wards. The progressive policy means that the challenge is met squarely through preventive measures in the community and intensive treatment in the hospital, and that many more of our citizens will be restored to a normal and productive life.

Broadly speaking, there are five types of administrative machines that have been set up in this country. It will be profitable to look at each form of control and discuss its strengths and weaknesses. In general they fall into two main groups: [18]

1. Supervision by full-time paid boards.
2. Supervision by volunteer boards.

1. *Supervision of all State correctional and charitable institutions by a paid control board.*

This is a form of organization adopted by many states where the small population renders many institutions unnecessary. The board has the supervision of all institutions—penal, correctional, insane, feebleminded, and epileptic. In a few states it has control over county and private hospitals. The membership is from three to five members, appointed by the Governor for a definite term. Occasionally the appointment is approved by the legislative body. In most states the membership is divided between the two dominant political parties. In a few states this control board consists of certain elective officers. The Governor is the chairman, and the treasurer and auditor are usually members. The law makes provision for a secretary and other office personnel. Such a board prescribes uniform record and accounting systems, appoints and discharges the chief executive officers and frequently other personnel, fixes salaries, purchases supplies, and has charge of the erection of new buildings and of all repairs and improvements. It supervises commitments and the discharge of patients.

The weaknesses of this form of organization are obvious. A board can never take the place of a responsible and well-trained executive. The method of appointment for a short term prevents any long-range planning. Policies cannot be continuous. The danger of appointments being political is great. In the administration of a highly intricate and technical phase of government such as the mental hospital represents, members of the control group must have special knowledge and experience to be efficient. A politically appointed board member transfers the interest and understanding of his own field to the problems of hospital management. If he is a farmer, the institution farm receives his attention; if a contractor, new building is his main interest; if a professional politician, more jobs. Such a control board can have little conception of the major problems involved in the prevention and treatment of mental illness.

It is impossible to hold the several members of a commission responsible for anything the group may do. Effective administration requires prompt decisions on multitudinous problems of day-to-day operation. When a board attempts to exercise administrative functions, it is practically certain that indecision and delays will be the rule. The necessary principle of board action that such decisions be unanimous makes such a situation unavoidable. Professional administration is practically a necessity for the efficient operation of any State mental hospital system.

2. *Supervision of all correctional and charitable institutions by an unpaid board of citizens.*

Members of the board are appointed by the Governor for a definite term. The number of members is from seven to ten. The term of office varies from two to seven years. The appointment of institutional heads, regular inspection, and the preparation of an annual report are part of the duties outlined by most of the statutes. In addition the board has the responsibility of deciding on standards of care and treatment, admission and discharge of patients, and the general welfare of the hospital population. Members receive only a *per diem* compensation for services actually rendered.

Here we have an example of amateur administration that is even more inefficient than the first form described. This system has all the faults of the paid board exaggerated to a greater degree. Such control board membership requires more time than any state has the right to ask a citizen to devote, if he is to give real service. The consideration of policies affecting the system must be carefully considered in the light of a full knowledge of the workings of the several institutional organizations. It would be impossible for such a board to acquire this information first hand. If the hospitals of any state are to be integrated towards a carefully thought out goal, there must be a coördinating head for the group. Without this, institutions develop a competitive spirit that cannot fail to interfere with that harmonious relationship which is essential if concerted action is to be achieved. There can be no uniformity of standards, and it becomes a race between executives to secure appropriations. Such tactics lead to unwise construction and unnecessary purchasing.

Political considerations invariably govern appointments to the board. Members are chosen because of party service and the institutions may become permeated by partisan politics. When this occurs the patients suffer. The uncertain tenure of office makes sustained policies impossible. Hospital administration is a specialty to which men should devote their entire lives. They formulate goals and policies which arise out of their experience and which are calculated to bring certain advantages to the patients. To subject these to a control board which is unsympathetic and un-understanding is to interfere seriously with the efficiency of the entire organization.

3. *No central control body. Supervision of each hospital by local boards of trustees or managers.*

Membership of these boards varies from three to ten. Members are usually appointed by the Governor for periods of from two to seven years. Election of the superintendent and other officers, regular visitation, and the preparation of an annual report comprise part of their functions. Such boards are frequently charged with a direct financial responsibility and inevitably they become interested in the problems of administration.

In this plan of operation there is even less efficiency than in either of the previously discussed systems. Each board and superintendent depends upon the political prestige of members for preferment in appropriation matters. The executive occupies himself with outside activities in order to get what money he needs, and in doing so is compelled to neglect the more important duties which relate to the administration of the institution. Each hospital being an independent unit, he thinks only in terms of his own local situation. He cannot see the problems from the state-wide point of view. It is rare to find a psychiatrist on any of these boards, and seldom do we find a member who has had any experience in mental hygiene. There are hundreds of splendid men and women on hospital boards in this country, serving without reward except for their own satisfaction, giving freely of their time and energy, trying to carry on a work for which they have had no training and in which they have had no experience. The formulation of general policies is an important function of any supervisory board, but administrative details are best carried on by one executive head.

4. *All institutions organized under a department of welfare with a division for each special group.*

Here we find a professional administration. The executive head of the department is a full-time commissioner appointed by the Governor for a definite term, which is usually from three to four years. He is experienced in some phase of social welfare. The department is organized into divisions, each of which is under an assistant commissioner who has had experience in the work he is to do. There are invariably divisions of correction, charity, mental hygiene, and child placing, each dealing with a particular phase of social welfare.

With this type of organization the state secures a better and more economical administration than could possibly be the case where unpaid or politically appointed paid boards are in control. A weakness of the plan is the fact that the term of office for which the director is appointed is too short to carry out long-time policies. The necessity for frequent reappointment makes it imperative that the commissioner spend more time than he should on outside matters. This is particularly true of states where the party in power changes frequently. Security for the executive head of the system is essential for true efficiency. Practically, this plan gives excellent results in the states where it has been in operation.

5. *Organization under a department of mental health with a full-time commissioner who is responsible for all mental hospitals, epileptic colonies, and schools for the feebleminded.*

Such a plan is practicable only where there is a sufficiently large population to necessitate many mental institutions. The outstanding examples of this type of organization are New York and Massachusetts. The law creating a department of mental health is similar in the two states except for minor details. New York has a state hospital commission consisting of three members. One of these must be a physician with at least ten years' general experience and five years in a mental institution. All of the commissioners are paid officials. They are appointed by the Governor—the medical commissioner during good behavior and the remaining two for six years.

The Massachusetts law provides that the commissioner of the Department of Mental Diseases must be a physician who has had experience in the care and treatment of mental patients. He is appointed for a term of five years. There are four associate commissioners, two of whom must be physicians experienced in the care and treatment of mental patients. The associate commissioners serve without pay except for a *per diem* compensation.

These states have set up in the statutory law protective provisions which insure skilled administration by trained people. The provision of the New York law that the medical commissioner must have actual mental hospital experience makes it stronger than the Massachusetts statute, which designates "experience in the care and treatment of mental patients." It would be better if the experience were more clearly defined. The New York law eliminates the specific term of office for the medical commissioner. This permits long-time policies to be put into effect. There can be a continuity to the administration which is impossible where a definite term is designated.

One of the important effects of such a system is that a promotional plan for personnel can be set up. Assistant physicians become eligible for assistant superintendencies and finally become executive heads of hospitals. The same line of advancement holds good in all departments. Every member of the hospital organization has ample opportunity to progress in his chosen field, and the constant movement of personnel makes promotion rapid. Both states have an excellent pension system, which in itself is an attraction and provides security.

A second advantage of this type of administration is that

coördination is possible. The entire mental hospital service becomes an integrated body and the effect upon the situation of such a mass approach should eventually bring results in the form of decreased admission and increased discharge rates. It is a sympathetic and understanding control. The practical experience of the commissioner is the greatest asset of the system. He knows the problems of the hospitals, understands their difficulties, and is able to bring the entire resources of the department into play for the purpose of inaugurating uniform standards of care and treatment.

The creation of a special department under the direction of a hospital-trained and experienced psychiatrist is the desirable form of state mental hospital administration. But there are smaller states where the problem is not so great as it is on the thickly populated Eastern seaboard. In such situations the organization of a department of welfare should be an efficient way of handling the problem. Such a department should be headed by a commissioner who would be appointed by the Governor from a list of at least three properly qualified individuals submitted by the board itself. There should be no restrictions on State residence, but outstanding men with records of actual achievement as administrators in this field should be secured wherever possible. The tenure of this office should be indefinite during meritorious service but with a provision that he may be removed for a sufficient cause by the Governor, after a hearing before the board of welfare. The director should be responsible to the Governor, the chief executive of the State. The salary should not be set by statute but provided in the current appropriation acts, and it must be sufficient to attract the best men. Welfare administration must be organized on a basis that will enable men to train for a career in that field. When we do this, the problems of mental disease, crime, and poverty will be nearer a satisfactory solution than they are today.

The board of welfare should preferably have a membership of not more than five, to be appointed by the Governor. There should be overlapping terms. It should be specifically stated in the law that appointments to this board must be made on the basis of demonstrated interest and familiarity with social welfare problems from the lay point of view and without regard to political affiliations or religious beliefs. The board should function as a policy-determining, rule-making, fact-finding, and advisory body. The members should receive no fixed salary but a compensation for actual duties performed.

The organization of such a department into divisions, each of which would be headed by an assistant director who is an authority in his special duties, would give the technical knowledge that is essential in this kind of administration. The number and character of these divisions would depend upon the local situation, but all of them should be under the control of the commissioner. Suggested divisions would be:

1. *Division of Mental Hygiene.* This division would be responsible for the entire program for the prevention and treatment of mental disease and health.

INSTITUTIONAL

a. Medical and Psychiatric Work
b. Psychiatric Nursing

EXTRA-INSTITUTIONAL

a. Social Service
b. Mental Clinics
c. Family Care

2. *Division of Correction.* This division would be responsible for all matters pertaining to the prisons and correctional institutions.

INSTITUTIONAL

a. Care and Treatment of Prisoners
b. Medical and Psychiatric Work
c. Industrial Management
d. Classification

EXTRA-INSTITUTIONAL

a. Probation
b. Parole

3. *Division of Charities.* Responsible for all institutional and extra-institutional charitable organizations.

a. Children's Homes
b. Child Placement and Guardianship

4. *Division of Public Health.* Responsible for all matters pertaining to the health of the citizens and the prevention of physical disease.

INSTITUTIONAL

a. Tuberculosis Hospitals
b. State Infirmary
c. Cancer Hospitals

EXTRA-INSTITUTIONAL

a. Pre-natal Care
b. Immunology
c. Epidemiology

5. *Division of Administration.* Responsible for all business matters pertaining to the department.

a. Central Accounting
b. Purchases and Stores
c. Establishment of Standards
d. Food Service
e. Plant Operation and Equipment
f. New Construction
g. Farms
h. Support

6. *Division of Statistics.* Responsible for the compilation of statistics from all departments for administrative control of operations and continuous planning.

a. Business
b. Psychiatric
c. Correctional
d. Charity
e. Health

Another type of organization which would make for efficiency in the smaller states would be to organize the entire mental hospital system under the Board of Health. The separation of mental hygiene from general health is not always for the best interest of the citizens.

HOSPITAL ORGANIZATION

The individual hospital tends to reflect the organization or lack of organization of the state in which it is located. Where there is a professional state administration, men are trained for positions of responsibility. But where there is loose organization with little or no coördination, the individual hospital frequently becomes a football for partisan politics and men are appointed to superintendencies without experience or training beyond a general medical education. They are, no doubt, conscientious individuals trying to do the job to the best of their ability, but frequently without the background which makes for efficiency.

American industry has pointed the way for hospital administration. Early in its development it became clear that efficient management was an indispensable factor in organization. Industrial leaders have insisted that a man who has been thoroughly trained in a special line of business and has shown characteristics that stamp him as a leader is cheap at any price. He is the one to promote business and safeguard industrial interests. But government has rarely applied this lesson to the administration of its departments. Men have been appointed to positions as superintendents of mental hospitals at salaries that a first-class mechanic would scorn, and yet these men have been charged with the responsibility of supervising costly plants and what is more important, human lives. Mental hospital administration should offer a career for which a man has to go through the most rigorous kind of training and for which he should receive substantial financial recognition for successful accomplishment.

Psychiatric organization has undergone many changes during the past two decades. The broadening of interests, the entrance into the field of representatives of other disciplines, and the participation of the institution in community affairs have created problems which are complex and confusing. The addition to staffs of highly specialized individuals has added to the problems of the administrator. Considering these facts, it is more essential than ever that proper standards be set up.

The final criterion for judging any hospital is a simple one. In the main the measures of achievement are:

1. Number of recovered patients being returned to the community.

2. Length of time these patients have spent in the hospital.
3. Length of time they remain in the community.

Fine buildings, good equipment, adequate records, and all the things we associate with well-managed hospitals are essential but unless they eventually lead to an increase in the discharge rate, shortening the hospital residence, and lengthening the time the patient spends in the community, the increased cost to the taxpayer is not justified.

What is a good mental hospital? Have we any standards by which such an institution may be measured? Hospitals have distinct personalities. This characteristic atmosphere can be detected by the trained observer the moment he steps into the entrance hall. It is as individual and marked as the architecture of the buildings or the plan of the grounds distinguishing one hospital from another. This personality pattern is set largely by the type of organization. And this in turn is the reflection of the chief executive. His personality governs the kind of organization, and the type of administration sets the emotional tone of the institution.

Broadly speaking, there are certain forms of administration. By this I mean the methods and techniques by which the plants are operated. There is the one-man type of administration, which is the traditional form in mental hospitals. The superintendent is the fountainhead of all ideas, orders, rules, methods, techniques, and procedures. A patient develops appendicitis. The administrator is the only one who may give permission for surgery. And the patient may die while he is being located or while he is revolving in his mind the possible legal entanglements which may ensue if the operation is not successful. Cautious conservatism usually goes hand in hand with this form of organization. It is essentially an absolute monarchy. Such an executive loads himself with a thousand details of management which would be more efficiently taken care of by assistants. He makes the decisions for everyone. When he leaves, the whole place stands still. His assistants are "yes men" and order-takers. When the load finally becomes so heavy that he staggers under it, his health suffers. Or the institution may function, stagnant and dead, with a routine custodial care meted out to patients.

This kind of organization does not develop men. It does not stimulate them to broader vision. It is rule by edict, discipline through fear which frequently grows out of the emotional instability and conflict of the head of the organization. The participation of others in his councils is a threat to his security. Such a system does not produce efficient hospital administration. It is only out of security that poise comes. The power of the mental hospital executive over his organization should be a sufficient compensation for him. The fact that he is conscious of this power should enable him to be tolerant and understanding in his relationships with those upon whom he depends.

Another type of hospital administration which has been tried is the dual-headed organization. Working on the theory that the institution has the double function of medical practice and business management, a few states have tried the experiment of placing a medical director in charge of the treatment of patients and a business manager in control of the economic side of the organization. This is an administrative absurdity, since such dual-headed forms of organization violate the major premise of good administration—one responsible head to every activity.

For many years the idea that physicians are not good business men has been prevalent. That a certain amount of justification for this view can be found is probably true. But to generalize the matter by saying that because of his medical education or perhaps because of the personality characteristics that impelled him to become a physician he is *per se* a failure in economic matters is the sheerest nonsense. A medical education should be a requirement for any hospital administrator. It is only through this background that he can apply the true principle of mental hospital administration, which is the cure of patients and the study and prevention of disease. With such an executive the values are medical rather than economic. With a business man with authority equal to that of the medical director and in control of financial expenditures, there is no question as to who sets the policies of the organization. In order to carry out the highest psychiatric ideals the medical executive must have financial control.

Finally there is the type of mental hospital organization of which this book is an advocate, a participative democracy. It is the intellectual freedom which permits free discussion and expression of opinion, out of which come new methods and avenues of approach. It is the synthesis of the ideas of many people into new formulations and policies. It is the way of progress. The psychiatric executive who closes his mind to the suggestions of his group is cutting off a rich source of stimulation for himself.

Emerson [14] says that there have always been two organization types. These he distinguishes as functional and military. The former is an organization to build up, the latter an organization to destroy. If one man uses the group to satisfy his own ego satisfaction, there can be little integration. And without this we get inefficiency. When all parts of the organization function as a whole and travel towards a common goal, we then arrive at the point where the group really makes progress. Throughout this book runs the thread of the argument—that the executive must ever be on the alert to harmonize the personal goal of his followers with the purpose of the organization. And the best way to formulate such common purposes is through group thinking and discussion.

One of the important principles of organization upon which Emerson laid great stress is the purpose of the group. Exactly what is the leader trying to achieve? The superintendent of a mental hospital who honestly asks himself this question may find himself in an embarrassing mental state. At first he will be hard put to evolve any answer beyond a vaguely general one. But if he perseveres and continues to think about it, he will probably find that he has more purposes than he has been consciously aware of. And when he gets the opinions of others in the group, he will be able to formulate something which can actually be given to everyone in the organization. What, then, should be the ideal of the psychiatric hospital? What are its functions? Exactly what is its place in the scheme of things? What will be its place twenty-five years from now? Should it be a passive agency, taking the patients sent to it, or should it be active and aggressive, reaching out to prevent the mental ills of the community? Are our methods satisfactory? If changes should be made, what are they and how should they be carried out? These and many other questions must be answered by the administrator who is thinking in terms of purpose.

Functional organization is built around the services for which the group is organized. Therefore, before any such organization can be built the executive must know what functions should be carried out. The thought on this point will range within wide limits. There will be as many opinions given as there are administrators. I have thought about the functions of a mental hospital as being primarily the five following:

1. *Practice of Psychiatry.* The progressive hospital will be receptive to new thought that is sound. It will be receptive even to those whose ideas are unusual, since psychiatry is in a nascent state and what is strange today may be commonplace tomorrow. It will open its ears and mind to the newer developments, studying them with a healthy skepticism but always requiring actual demonstration. It will be ready to open the door to the representatives of other social sciences who may have contributions to make. The problems of mental disease will never be solved by one professional group working alone. Coordination and coöperation are essential if further progress is to come. If we as physicians elect to assume a "holier-than-thou" attitude in this matter it might be well to recall a statement of that talented physician, great humanitarian, and splendid gentleman, Oliver Wendell Holmes.[15] "Medicine learned," said he, "from a Jesuit how to cure agues, from a friar how to cut for the stone, from a soldier how to treat gout, from a sailor how to keep off scurvy, from a postmaster how to sound the Eustachian tube, from a dairymaid how to prevent smallpox, and from an old woman how to catch the 'itch insect.' " There are so many examples that to recapitulate them might result in our becoming too humble. The important point is that the administrator can well afford to maintain a receptive attitude towards the disciplines allied to psychiatry. Progress is probably in that direction.

2. *Medicine and Surgery.* The somatopsychic relationship is receiving much attention from thoughtful physicians. In our eagerness to uncover subconscious conflicts and obscure emotional entanglements, we must not forget that there is a body

involved in the situation, the exact relationship of which to the psyche is not known. The practice of sound medicine and surgery will inspire respect and increase prestige. Therefore we must list medicine and surgery as a function of the mental hospital.

3. *Teaching.* The teaching hospital is the best type of institution. It gives patients better care and has higher scientific standards than the institution which has no educational program. The dissemination of health knowledge extramurally is also a responsibility of every hospital. Even though the individual who receives training in psychiatry never specializes in that field, he goes into the community with a better conception of psychiatric problems and what is being done to solve them. He is a liaison officer who can interpret the organization to society and help create a better understanding of the functions of the hospital.

4. *Research.* Certainly one of the functions of the mental hospital must be psychiatric research. For a hundred years we have been trying to solve the problems of mental disease by building more buildings to house more patients. No state has ever been able to meet the constantly increasing demands. The cry of "overcrowding" goes on continually, and we are in a condition of confusion most of the time. Does it not seem reasonable to pause in the mad scramble for new construction and consider whether there is some other approach to a solution of the problem? Research in psychiatry is far behind, and the sooner a mass attack is made to get at the cause of mental disease instead of just describing it, the sooner we shall begin to make an impression on the growing load of cases.

5. *Prevention.* The mental hospital must accept some responsibility for the mental health of its community. Preventive psychiatry offers as much hope for the future as does preventive medicine. Educational efforts are a part of a mental hygiene program. Clinics for both children and adults are a part of this same movement. The psychiatric institution must prepare itself to carry on both. Preventive psychiatry must be considered as an essential function of the mental hospital.

With these functions in mind, I offer a statement of purpose for the mental hospital administrator to consider as a goal.

A. To bring about a perceptible decrease in the incidence of mental disorder in the general community.
   1. By rendering a real service to the community and making the hospital a place to which individuals turn for a settlement of their troubles and difficulties.
   2. By enlisting the people of the State in this campaign and getting them to share the responsibility by a better understanding of the problem of mental disorders.
   3. By disseminating information about mental health and disease as rapidly as it is accumulated and teaching people the preventive aspects of these disorders.
   4. By developing the hospital as a research center and making a substantial contribution to the sum total of our knowledge of the etiology, prevention, and treatment of mental disease.
   5. By enlarging the present clinic facilities in the community for the study and treatment of adults and children who show abnormal behavior reactions.

B. To discharge more patients into the community, to decrease the time spent by each patient in the hospital, and to increase the time spent outside by those who may have to return.
   1. By constantly keeping before each member of the organization the true measure by which individual efficiency is to a considerable extent judged—i.e., the recovery of patients.
   2. By making continuous efforts to integrate the entire group towards this common goal.
   3. By thinking always in terms of human beings instead of bricks and mortar.
   4. By making the administrative routine of the hospital a therapeutic factor which is concerned primarily with the recovery of the patient and the prevention of mental disease.

C. To make the hospital a center of activity for all who may have an interest in the mental problems of human beings.
   1. By welcoming all sound new thought in psychiatry.

2. By inviting representatives of the social sciences and other disciplines to utilize the facilities of the hospital and permitting them to make such contributions to the program as may be possible.
3. By constantly exemplifying the fact that the sensible approach to the problems of psychiatry is a coördinated one—a matter of teamwork.

D. To indicate the contribution psychiatry has to make to general medicine.
1. By carrying on a teaching program for medical students and graduates which is designed to show that the illnesses of human beings are mental as well as physical.
2. By teaching general nurses that the patient is a human being as well as a case.
3. By carrying on a high type of medical and surgical work and contributing facts regarding the relationship between the psyche and the soma.

E. To carry out these purposes with due consideration for the economic cost and with the rights of the community constantly in mind.
1. By keeping the costs of the hospitals as low as is consistent with the type of service needed to carry out this program.
2. By constantly utilizing new ideas, from whatever source they may come, in efforts to lower the costs of such service.
3. By endeavoring to get State governments to see that the real solution of the problem lies in personnel rather than in buildings.

There need be no rigidity about the goal but there must be some legitimate purpose which can be clearly formulated for the members of the organization. The administrator must keep in mind the necessity for adjusting the individual goal to the purpose of the institution. And here it may be necessary to set up certain minor goals for those groups who work best for a purpose that can be attained more quickly. If the purpose of the individual is to obtain financial reward, he cannot wait until this broad general goal has been attained. Consequently a minor purpose which depends upon personal effort must be set up, and when that goal is reached, financial reward should come. The goal of the individual may be power, social approval, or recognition by an individual or group to whom he is loyal. To carry out this principle each department director must know his employees intimately. In order to direct men and women along these lines, one must know their background, their capabilities, their motives, and what they hope to attain. The day will eventually come when the mental hospital will take another lesson from industry and utilize the services of a well-trained personnel director. Such an officer, not being in authority over the employee, would be able to know more about him than one who regulated his life.

Whatever the plan of organization, it should be definitely known to the entire group. The wall charts which are used by executives in industry indicate the lines of authority and responsibility. There should be no confusion in the mind of anyone about these relationships. A copy of this organization chart should hang in every office so that department heads might call the attention of each new employee to it and instruct older workers regarding promotion possibilities. This is one of the devices by which coördination of the group is attained.

Paper plans are of no value, however, unless they are carried out in practice. I have known cases where elaborate wall charts were prepared and yet in the functioning of the hospital few members of the organization knew what their authority was and to whom they were responsible. It is through these contacts that the superintendent coördinates and correlates the work of professional and lay workers. Whatever plan of operation is used, it should be worked out to fit the needs of the particular institution and should be more than a blue print hanging on the wall.

Inasmuch as there is a distinct line of demarcation between the professional and business sides of the institution, the simple plan of organization would be to have a steward in charge of the business operations and a clinical director responsible for all professional activities. Each would deal directly with the superintendent or assistant superintendent. This is the scheme of operation in a number of psychiatric institutions. The advantages of such a simple type of organization are that it narrows the number of individuals with whom the executive has to deal and definitely fixes responsibility. It decreases the danger of friction between department heads and permits work to be planned more efficiently and economically.

The plan has disadvantages, however. The small number of people who come into contact with the superintendent lessens his field of direct influence. The coördinating power between business and professional activities is in the hands of the superintendent and he alone can bring these two groups together. While it is an efficient scheme of organization, it does not give the best results from the standpoint of improved morale.

A preferable plan would be to divide the entire hospital into departments, each being under the direction of a responsible head who would report directly to the superintendent. These department heads would form the professional and lay councils that advise the executive on matters of importance. A list of such departments would include psychiatric, engineering, maintenance, farm, steward, and treasurer.

Hospital psychiatry is the most conspicuous example of State medicine to be found in the United States. It has been accepted for many years by the medical profession because the problem of mental disease is too vast for any other agency to cope with successfully. Because of the complexity of the problem, efficient professional State administration is essential if patients are to be treated and cured rather than held in custody. Lay boards, paid or unpaid, furnish only amateur leadership and do not serve the best interests of the taxpayer or the sick individual. Partisan politics, which interfere with hospital administration and particularly personnel selection, cannot be condemned too strongly. When political considerations enter the hospital, professional efficiency flies out of the window. And frequently even good custodial care accompanies it. Mental hospital administration calls for qualities of leadership, psychiatric knowledge, and executive ability that can be gained only by experience. But even these qualities are of no value unless the executive is free from selfish and unskillful interference.

The traditional type of administration has been found to be unprofitable by industry, and the administrator will find it worth while to consider seriously a more democratic plan of organization. The coördination of the group is his chief concern. The hospital functions, to a considerable extent, in accordance with the personality of the executive. If he has emotional poise and mental security, he will build his organization around that plan which best develops the members of the group into more efficient individuals who are capable, because of this experience, of advancing to greater responsibilities.

Chapter 3

BUILDING A STAFF

In any discussion of staff organization, two phases of administration must receive consideration, and every hospital executive decides questions of policy largely on the basis of one or the other, depending upon where he places his values. On the one hand there is the professional group, which concerns itself with matters of diagnosis, treatment, and research; on the other hand there are those members of the organization whose chief responsibilities are financial and economic. The one who must maintain the balance between these essential types of activities is the superintendent. It is he who places the emphasis upon one or the other and thus establishes the general atmosphere of the institution. This atmosphere may indicate that the major interests of the hospital are either professional or economic. If the former, the visitor feels in those with whom he comes in contact an enthusiasm for therapy, research, and teaching. On the other hand, this atmosphere may indicate that the main interest is economic. In this case he hears only discussions about low per capita costs, fine cattle, fertile fields, and other material considerations. The executive is largely responsible for this institutional attitude.

The thesis of this chapter is that the professional group must be the dominant one in the psychiatric organization if it is to function as a hospital and not as a business with the professional activities incidental. The leadership of the institution must be professional if it is to be a healing agency. That the business side is important no one will deny. The economic factor will always affect scientific considerations. Quantity of production must always be kept in relationship with financial possibilities. It may not be possible to do as much psychiatric research as one desires because sufficient money is not available, but certainly the quality of the professional work is subject to no such limitation. There may be too few physicians on the staff, but this is no legitimate reason why the administrator should not get the best ones to be had and hold them to a high level of professional performance. Insufficient money for medical work may be available, but what is accomplished should be of the highest standard. In a hospital where scientific and educational ideals are the major interests, business considerations will always give way to medical and psychiatric needs. If a choice must be made between an expenditure for the farm and a psychiatric necessity, the far-seeing administrator will give the professional requirement precedence.

Financial security is not the first requisite to hospital progress. The desire and enthusiasm for progressive change must always come first. The executive who waits to inaugurate a research program in his hospital until ample funds are available will probably never take the first step. The inculcation of the spirit to do must always be preliminary to any action, and when this attitude becomes the dominant one in the organization, the force of group enthusiasm leads to obtaining some financial support.

To discuss the qualifications which are essential for the executive head of a mental hospital is to open up the whole subject of the psychology of leadership. Autocratic administration has been the rule in many psychiatric institutions. Superintendents have used the old militaristic methods which came from early American industry, where authority flowed directly from the boss to the men. Modern industrial management has discovered that a more democratic type of organization produces better results. Integrated working spirit does not generate spontaneously but only in direct proportion to the constructive type of leadership given. The inculcation of a harmonious, willing, and loyal *esprit de corps* in a complex and complicated organization such as that of a mental hospital calls for the very highest type of executive leadership. The administrator must be a teacher, a leader, a stimulator, a coordinator, and a developer of younger men.

Mental hospital executives have been rather slow to adopt these newer theories of management. Psychiatrists have not hesitated to apply their formulations to the problems of industrial management. They have been willing to advise the business man about his difficulties with employees, but apparently these principles have escaped our attention when dealing with the same questions in our psychiatric hospitals. Should we not therefore study our executive procedures to see if the leadership we are giving is based upon sound psychological policies?

Tead [16] defines leadership as "the integration of the activities of an entire group towards the particular goal which is desired by all." Integration means in management exactly what it means in psychology, bringing the parts into action as one harmonious whole. Therefore the problem of the administrator is the integration of his working group towards a common goal which has been set up. "Leadership is that combination of qualities by the possession of which one is able to get something done by others, because through his influence, they desire to do it." A portion of this definition should be emphasized—"because through his influence, they desire to do it." True leadership is active, not passive. The executive molds his people and influences their thoughts, desires, and actions.

Tead further states:—

"The elements, first, of a definite objective and, second, of influencing people so that their own desires harmonize with those of the leader, are both essential. It is this which is creative leadership, as distinct from ways of getting people to act which do not take their desires into account. The new and distinguishing element is the creation and direction of positive desire in the led. Something over and above mere consent is implied. It means actually taking over as one's very own the purpose of the leader. Or, more fundamentally, it implies the evoking by the leader and the led together of new reaches of purpose, the realizing of which is discovered by all to bring about a more effective fulfillment of the desires of all."

This, if applied to the hospital superintendent, places an entirely different construction on his responsibilities. Instead of making him a boss who issues authoritative edicts for others to obey, it puts up to him squarely the question of seeking to know the desires of those he is directing and trying to adapt these desires to the goal of the group. Every executive is a leader. His task is to be the builder of a group animated by satisfying, common purposes. Every staff physician, department head, head nurse, and attendant is a leader.

While hospital administrative methods can to some extent be acquired, there is unfortunately no school which teaches them. The only way in which the young physician can secure training is to serve an apprenticeship of many years. Out of this experience he attempts to formulate a philosophy of management. What he becomes eventually is largely dependent upon the ability and willingness of the man under whom he serves to teach him general principles and permit him to devise his own techniques. Because of the tendency of executives to pass on methods and systems instead of general policies, we frequently see the apprentice become a pocket edition of his preceptor.

To give the type of creative leadership which results in an integrated working spirit, the administrator should have certain characteristics. Some of these are natural traits which may be further developed by training and experience. Others can never be acquired. No man possesses all the qualifications that go to develop complete efficiency in his organization. But no man can give the kind of leadership which makes for psychiatric progress who cannot convey to his followers certain qualities that weld all elements of the group together. He must be able to give to those about him a strength and power which stimulate each to maximum efforts in progressing towards the goal that has been set.

Such a leader will apply his psychiatric knowledge of the emotional lives of human beings to his administrative problems. He will use this understanding to vary his techniques in accordance with the personality of the individual. He will be tolerant of the intellectual opinions of others, and while he will always be ready to make the final decision and accept the responsibility of these decisions, he will, when possible, divide this responsibility with his partners.

Enthusiasm, imagination, and initiative are essential qualities of this type of executive. The pessimistic, "What's the use!" superintendent cannot stimulate his organization to any great extent. The characteristic that enables him to think faster than others gives confidence to those who work with him. The ability to visualize a plan which may take years to mature, to take the data of past experience and apply them in newly conceived combinations, is an essential trait for the creative leader.

Courage and persistence are necessary. The superintendent who is too timid and fearful to strike out into untrodden fields will find his organization in a state of stagnation. Hospitals are in a constant state of flux. The need for courage is clearly indicated in the extraordinary conditions that have prevailed during the past years. The executive who gives up at the first rebuff and fails to surmount obstacles that are placed in his path will have to develop this trait if he is to provide creative leadership.

The executive who has a clear-cut idea of the purposes of his organization has gone a long way towards constructive leadership. He must believe in these purposes so unremittingly that he works for them constantly. One may have purposes, but unless they can be translated into accomplishments they are of little value. He who reflects upon the wisdom of his purposes is a philosopher rather than a leader. Finally he must have a fair degree of confidence in himself. To have self-confidence does not mean that he fancies himself as an authority on every subject. It implies that he has a belief in certain principles and in his ability to carry them out, and is able to go on with a sense of security which permits him to fight for those things in which he believes.

The particular thing that distinguishes the creative executive is his attitude towards the group. He is sympathetic, tolerant, and understanding, and above all has an affection for them that impels him to think in terms of their interests as well as his own. The superintendent who sees a personal insult in the desire of his assistant to better himself by going to another hospital to gain additional experience will not go far in building an integrated unit.

THE PROFESSIONAL STAFF

The wisdom with which the administrator selects his professional and lay assistants is the most important indication of his executive ability. If he is satisfied with men whose only qualification is that they have a degree or laymen whose principal claim to advancement is that they have been in the service a certain length of time, he cannot hope to have a successful participating democracy. If he selects mediocre individuals, they will see in his attempts to delegate authority and responsibility only a desire to overwork them or a wish to evade his own responsibilities. His insistence that staff members make their own decisions in professional matters is apt to be interpreted as timidity. Such men do not respond to the stimulation that should come with the assumption of greater responsibility. They become querulous and fault-finding, and are critical of others who may see in the position more than a mere job.

A young and ambitious psychiatrist was considering an important position in a mental hospital organization where a democratic type of administration was in effect. To secure data upon which to base his decision, he interviewed two men, each of whom had been on the staff. One had left to accept a promotion, the other had gone to another institution without a change in status. In his attempt to get the reaction of both to the policies of the executive he received two different replies. The one in the higher position said, "By all means take the place. You will have an opportunity to assume as much responsibility as you wish. It is the best experience you can get." The second individual warned the psychiatrist not to accept the position "because he will make you do all the work."

SELECTING A STAFF

How can we attract to the mental hospital service the best trained men from medical and other professional schools? Is it possible to make psychiatry so interesting that they will find such a career worth while? These are the questions the administrator must answer if he wishes to build a self-reliant and loyal staff of ambitious and enthusiastic men and women. It is not always easy to find the proper reply. But each executive must find his own answers. Mental hospitals labor under the handicap of essentially treating chronic illnesses. The ambitious young physician can see no professional satisfaction in such practice. The medical schools have not always been helpful to the hospital. Psychiatric internships have not been made popular. Other professional schools have had a similar attitude. But above all, the attitude of the hospital itself has not always been calculated to attract the men who graduate in the upper third of their class. The isolation, both professional and social, the lack of psychiatric and medical activity, and the discipline under which some mental hospital staffs must work and live, have all tended to discourage ambitious young men and women from entering the field of psychiatry. Frequently the administrator does not have the privilege of selecting his own staff. Civil service rules may regulate the employment of professional people. Political expediency frequently governs the selection. Both of these methods are unsatisfactory from the standpoint of a well-integrated organization. The means by which the individual administrator will attract his staff will be different in each situation.

There are several factors which enter into the problem of staff selection that every hospital executive must seriously consider. I enumerate them in the order of their importance.

Medical and Psychiatric Activity

The hospital that is active medically and psychiatrically will always attract the best professional people. An atmosphere of this kind makes up for many deficiencies of other sorts. In such an institution high professional standards will prevail and the earnest student will welcome such a regime. Teaching, research, a wide variety of psychiatric thought, and an active medical and surgical service are all important factors in creating a professional tone that attracts competent staff members. Good psychiatric leadership is an essential. But above all the hospital must have intellectual freedom. It cannot be controlled by the traditions and prejudices of one individual. The right to think implies the right to disagree.

Suitable Living Conditions

Except for economic reasons, I can see no justification for a continuation of the policy of "living in" for staff members. I realize that local conditions may make it impossible to do otherwise, but wherever possible, professional men and their families should live in the community. Even if houses are provided, there is a constant temptation to narrow the field of interest to the hospital group. A cloistered existence of this kind is not mentally healthy. To live a contented home life one should be reasonably free from dictation in social and family relationships. This is not always possible in the close-knit hospital community.

Living outside the institution, the right kind of professional staff, through their social contacts, would add immeasurably to the prestige of the hospital. They would interpret its work to a greater number of thinking people, and their influence in their own social group could not help but be beneficial.

The economic argument has been raised with regard to "living in." Whether the system really saves money is a debatable point. When the cost of construction and maintenance is considered, it is doubtful whether a real saving is effected by giving family maintenance as a part of the salary. Where conditions render it necessary for professional staff members to live on the hospital grounds, the accommodations should be suitable for well-educated and cultured people.

SALARY

The question of salary is one that will always be controlled by the law of supply and demand. If we are to attract and retain well-trained men of ability in the psychiatric hospital service, we must seriously consider this question. Consideration must be given to the creation of higher positions in the service to which young clinicians may aspire. As the matter now stands, the psychiatrist who is interested in clinical psychiatry finds his way to the higher positions cut off. He can secure no advancement except through the avenue of administration. If clinical directorships were the rule rather than the exception, they would furnish an outlet for ambitious clinical staff members.

PROMOTION

The executive who is looking for the best men for higher positions will, of course, turn to his own staff first. Long-continued service is not always for the best interest of either individual or hospital. A reasonably rapid turnover of the professional staff is healthy. New blood must be injected into the organization at intervals if it is to be virile and dynamic. The hospital that has the reputation of placing its men in better positions will always be attractive to young people of ability. Opportunity for reasonable advancement is an important factor. Promotion should be fairly rapid but must be based on meritorious work and not on mere length of service. To advance men into higher grades for the sentimental reason that they have served a certain length of time is poor administration. Promotions should come only as the result of outstanding contributions to the organization.

It is axiomatic in administration that every key man should have an understudy. Ideally there should never be a time when the superintendent does not have a man in training to step into the place of one higher in the organization. He selects and retains professional people only on the basis of their ability and fitness to be promoted. F. B. Gilbreth[17] advocated the "three position" plan of promotion. He believed that every man should belong to three groups. He is, at the same time, a worker, a teacher, and an apprentice. While working at his own job he is teaching a man from the group below him to take his place and at the same time is training himself in the duties of the group above him. He is promoted only when he is thoroughly familiar with the work of the position to which he is going and after he has trained someone to take his place. Such a plan should work well in a mental hospital. The senior physician trains the junior to take his place and at the same time is learning the duties of assistant superintendent or clinical director. But it is important that the selection and advancement of men depend upon definite measures of ability rather than upon the personality reaction and emotional prejudices of the administrator.

Can standards be devised that will give a fair estimate of the contribution of any individual? The industrial executive has production costs and financial return as measures of efficiency. But the gauge of psychiatric ability is less clearly defined. The discharge of patients is certainly one of the ways by which the worth of the staff member may be determined. If the psychiatrist is to be more than a supervisor, he must get results in the form of improved and recovered patients. The ability to write well-phrased ward notes or diagnostic summaries of literary merit is well enough, but unless there is an urge to utilize such ability in actual patient therapy it is of little value. The agreeable, popular ward psychiatrist may not be of assistance in advancing the organization towards the goal.

To check and measure the usefulness of any psychiatrist is the constant aim of the responsible superior. He judges each man at frequent intervals by getting complete information on characteristics such as the following:

1. TECHNICAL SKILL

A. *Psychiatry*

What is his interest in psychiatry?

Has he a constructive psychiatric point of view, or is he merely a note-writer?

Does he know and utilize all of the resources of the hospital in the application of psychiatry to his patients?

How well does he know his patients?

Is he a student and does he read to perfect his knowledge?

Is he able to write good case records and can he present them at staff conference?

Are his discussions and comments in staff meeting worthy of attention?

B. *Medicine and Surgery*

Is he alert to the necessity of the study of cases from the physical point of view?

Does he use the medical and surgical service as a psychiatric aid, or does he pass patients along and give no further thought to them?

Does he keep in touch with his patients on the medical service?

Do his notes show an interest in medical matters?

Does he attend and take part in autopsies and clinico-pathological conferences?

C. *Administration*

1. *Records*

Does he understand the significance of proper records, or are they made only because it is required?

Does he keep up his routine work or is it necessary to prod him constantly?

Do his notes show a real understanding of patients?

2. *Housekeeping*

Does he recognize the importance of good housekeeping as of psychiatric significance?

3. *Detail*

Does he handle details well?

Can he see administrative details from the standpoint of psychiatry?

2. PERSONAL GROWTH

Is he broadening his outlook?

Does he show a broadening interest in his profession and specialty?

Does he visit other hospitals to get new viewpoints?

Does he attend medical and psychiatric meetings?

Is he interested in trying to solve psychiatric problems through research?

Has he written any papers that are worth while?

3. HABITS

Is he industrious?

Does he bear his share of the load?

Does he organize his time intelligently?

Does he take sufficient recreation?

Does he have friends outside the hospital?

Is he interested in community affairs?

What are his relations with:

A. Visitors
B. Subordinates
C. Other staff members
D. Other departments
E. Students

Does he give up to the limit of his mental ability?

Is he optimistic towards the future of his specialty?
Is he loyal to the entire organization?
Is he persistent, in a quiet way, in getting his ideas across, or does he give up after one set-back?
Has he progressed beyond mere technical proficiency?

4. ABILITY TO ATTACK AND SOLVE A PROBLEM

Has he an understanding of the details of a situation?
Can he find a proper solution for problems presented?

5. INITIATIVE AND RESOURCEFULNESS

What has he suggested that has contributed towards the progress of the hospital?
Is he fertile in excuses and alibis?
Does he ever devise new ways of doing things or is he resistant to new ideas?
Is he resourceful in finding ways and means of meeting unusual situations?

6. CHARACTER QUALITIES

Has he sustained enthusiasm or is he inclined to plunge into things and then give them up easily?
Does he wait patiently for the proper time to do things or does he rush in without adequate preparation?

7. OUTLOOK

Has he the ability to see the immediate tasks?
Can he see the hospital in its broader relations to the community and is he willing to accept some of the responsibility for these relationships?

8. FUTURE PROSPECTS

Is he timber for further advancement?
Will he stop in his present position indefinitely?
Will he move fast enough to permit younger men to have their chance?
Will he accept the responsibility of teaching and training younger men?

This general scheme may be readily modified to fit other professional groups.

The practice of reviewing cases at the end of each year serves as another way of keeping a check on the performance of individual staff members. In a loose-leaf book the executive has a list of patients entering the hospital during the month. Twelve columns extend across the double page, each representing a month. On the first day of each month the secretary notes the ward on which the patient is at that time, and at the end of the year a complete record of the patient's progress through the hospital is before the superintendent. He makes use of it by asking each member of the staff to justify the further residence of every patient remaining.

If a patient has been on an open ward for several months, the question is raised as to what steps are being taken to get him home. Open ward patients get lost in the hospital. They are assigned to industrial positions, become efficient workers, and frequently bog down into an apathetic acceptance of the situation. Such patients should be forced out of the hospital before they settle into a groove.

The case of the patient who remains on a medical ward month after month should be reviewed. The cost of general hospital treatment is considerably higher than the expense of maintaining a patient on a psychiatric ward. A review of the therapy carried out will not infrequently reveal a failure to apply some procedure that would accelerate the recovery of the patient, physically, at least, if not psychiatrically. Careless medical practice should never be tolerated by the mental hospital administration. I have known a patient to be observed month after month with psychiatric records showing that somatic delusions were present. Finally a young physician full of enthusiasm and scientific curiosity arranged for an exploratory operation, and an extensive duodenal ulcer was found. This failure to investigate the somatic side of the problem is careless psychiatric practice.

When the patient has remained on a disturbed ward for an unusually long period, a review of the treatment may reveal that a change of environment is indicated or that a different type of ward administration is needed. Scrutiny of treatment methods is an excellent index of the efficiency of both psychiatrist and nurse. Physicians tend to lose interest in the patient who is actively disturbed over a long period of time. The nurse reflects the attitude of the psychiatrist. If he takes only a perfunctory interest in the matter, she is likely to adopt a similar attitude.

THE COUNCIL

Having secured a high-grade staff, it is essential that the executive consider carefully the kind of organization under which the group will work best. Such a staff does not ordinarily respond well to autocratic dictation. Individuals of high intellectual ability who are loyal to the ideals of the group will not willingly be repressed by traditional attitudes. They cannot be handled like children. Such men do not function well in an atmosphere of autocratic dictatorship, and the executive who tries to rule them with a high hand will find his staff continuously disintegrating. This kind of staff creates administrative problems that would not be present with a less able group, but the contribution they make to the hospital may outweigh these considerations.

Superintendents who wish to assume a real leadership and secure the highest possible type of loyalty will do well to set up the organization on democratic lines. Such a plan of administration involves more than mere majority control. A participating democracy goes further. Out of free discussion and interchange of opinion come entirely new plans that are accepted by the group. This does not mean that every person in the organization should have a voice in policy building. Lest someone get the idea that I am advocating a form of administration where the superintendent is only a member of the group and every man is equal, I hasten to disclaim any such intention. The essence of the superintendent's attitude is his willingness to accept advice—not to abrogate his authority.

Any modern organization will function more efficiently if the leader has at his command a body of expert knowledge to assist in creating suitable policies. With a qualified staff "he builds from the bottom instead of futilely dictating from the top." This modern type of organization is exemplified by the general staff of the United States Army. The staff is made up of specialists and experts in all fields, who bring to bear upon every problem all the expert knowledge obtainable. The medical council which meets regularly with the superintendent is comparable to the general staff of the army. It is organized for the purpose of discussing and formulating medical and psychiatric policies. All professional departments should be represented. The assistant superintendent, clinical director, chief of research, director of the outpatient clinic, chief psychologist, and director of the laboratories should be members. Such questions as the addition of new professional personnel, promotions to higher grades, nursing policies, financial matters, at least in so far as they relate to professional work, new equipment and construction as it affects patients, and research progress are all proper matters for discussion and settlement by the council.

But here a word of warning is necessary. The hospital executive who really wishes to use this plan must be prepared to follow the decisions of the group in fact. Merely to get them together to listen to a monologue by the "chief" is neither helpful nor morale-building. Unless one is prepared actually to abide by the conclusions of the council, he had better go on making his own decisions. Any attempt on the part of the executive to dominate the thoughts of men who are competent to sit in this council would be fatal to the plan.

The superintendent who sees in group decisions a loss of power cannot handle this type of organization successfully. When he closes his mind to the suggestions of assistants he loses a valuable means of building morale and increasing loyalty. The superintendent who replies to the suggestion of his assistant that a certain project be tried by saying, "I am the head of this institution. Your business is to carry out my orders. When I want this done I shall let you know," is not improving the loyalty of that assistant.

The psychiatric leader will seek the counsel of his cabinet to judge the abilities and fitness of new men. He will not rely entirely on his own judgment. While education, training, and cultural background are essential, personality and the ability to fit into the group are equally important. A harmonious working organization is made up of individuals of equal abilities, within limits, but also of those whose personalities mesh together.

The policy of permitting department heads of the professional staff to have a large part in the selection of their own colleagues brings rich returns in the form of better loyalty and closer coöperation with the policies of the hospital. When men have a real responsibility in the selection of those who work with them they will be careful to add to the staff only those who will reflect credit on their judgment. They feel the responsibility of making the relationship pleasant for the new staff member and assisting him in every way possible so that he may make his best contribution to the organization. This is partnership.

In order to make such decisions intelligently, the council must not only be informed of all the policies but must have had a share in their formulation. It is not safe to rely on the judgment of men who are working in the dark. They must have all the data for drawing conclusions that the executive himself possesses. The secretiveness of many administrators about their plans is not conducive to good morale.

Under such a system, decisions frequently are taken out of the hands of the superintendent. There is the instance of the request from the chief of the research division to purchase a rather expensive piece of equipment which was needed for a new project. The answer of the executive was, "Doctor, you know our financial situation as well as I do. If you say that we can buy this and save enough to pay for it out of the general fund for research, I shall be glad to approve the purchase. Please let me know when you make your final decision." Several days later the assistant informed the superintendent that he had decided not to purchase the equipment, because other things were needed that should take precedence over that particular article.

Committee Organization

To gain the coöperation of every member of the professional staff, each must have some share in forming plans and some part in devising methods of management. It is their knowledge, experience, and information about detail that will keep the administrator out of many difficulties. The use of committees in mental hospital administration is a further elaboration of the general staff idea. When organizations build their own routine, members are more apt to carry it out conscientiously than if a set of rules were handed to them. Every broad administrative problem which needs consideration can be referred to such a committee. For instance, why is the hospital having so many escapes? No one can answer this question. The autocratic superintendent goes into a tirade and issues numerous orders which are soon forgotten by everyone. The creative executive refers the question to a committee consisting of a senior and junior physician from each service. A questionnaire is devised by the committee and each patient who returns from escape is interrogated along the lines indicated in the questionnaire. After a study of fifty escapes, a new standard practice is evolved to take care of the situation, and incidentally, a great deal of psychiatric material is secured which is of value in other administrative departments.

The linen inventories show a greater loss in sheets than they should. The superintendent could fly into a rage, reprimand everyone in sight, and throw the whole organization into a turmoil. Instead he appoints a committee consisting of the assistant superintendent, the director of nursing, and the matron to investigate the matter. The committee report locates the source of the difficulty and a new standard practice is recommended to cover the weak points.

Still again, staff meetings are becoming a bore. They cease to be interesting. What is the difficulty? A committee consisting of the senior physician on each of three services and the chief psychologist is appointed. They study the situation and make a report which embodies an entirely new plan of case presentation to the staff. After free discussion the principles of the recommendation are accepted and become standard practice.

Standing committees which have a fixed membership and function in certain routine matters are of great value. If there is a training school in the hospital, a committee should be an integral part of it. The school committee might include the clinical director, chief psychologist, director of laboratories, director of research, director of nursing, instructors, etc. All matters pertaining to the school are brought before this committee. They consider the qualifications of students, passing grades, advise as to curriculum, and study training school policies. A standing committee should meet at regular intervals. A committee to consider and regulate the combined teaching in all departments is of inestimable value. The clinical director is chairman of this group. Members will be those heads of divisions in which teaching is carried on, e.g., the head social worker, head occupational therapist, director of nurses, pathologist, chief psychologist. The committee has the responsibility of considering general teaching activities. A personnel committee should be responsible for grading the work of ward employees and considering promotions. Membership might consist of the assistant superintendent, the senior physician of each service, the director of nurses, and each chief supervisor.

In carrying through the idea of democracy, a committee to consider disciplinary problems among employees should be in existence instead of permitting ward personnel to be at the mercy of the whims of one individual. It is better to have these matters decided by a group. Such a group could consist of the superintendent, assistant superintendent, director of nurses, senior physician, chief supervisor, and assistant supervisors of the service on which the offending individual is employed.

The question as to the desirability of spending the time necessary for these committees may be raised. Practically, it will be found that the total time spent by any one individual, with the possible exception of the superintendent, is not excessive. There should be a division of labor for two reasons. The greater the number who participate in these committee activities, the better will be the effect on morale. The more people who participate, the less burden each will have to carry. In one hospital the nurses' and attendants' homes were managed by house committees which recommended improvements, took care of minor infractions of its rules, looked after the homes, and generally took the responsibility of matters in that department. The virtue of the committee system is that it insures coöperation on the part of the minor executives and turns them into the path of real leadership. Committees foster a spirit of loyalty and partnership, convey the ideas of the administration to followers because of the closer association of the members, and finally build a group spirit, the like of which could never be attained under an autocratic regime.

In his attempts to mold the desires of men, the administrator will afford his staff opportunity to inform themselves about what he is trying to accomplish. He will not be secretive about his aims. His plans for the future will be well known, partly because he disseminates the information and partly because they are the result of group deliberation. He will meet his staff at regular intervals for the discussion of purely administrative topics which have a bearing upon the therapy of patients. An hour each week can well be devoted to such staff meetings. Committee reports and general topics may also be brought up for discussion. A monthly quantitative analysis of the psychiatric and medical work of the hospital should be presented regularly. It might cover in detail the entire professional work of the institution, showing the movement of population, the admissions, discharges, and types of commitment, and including a report from every professional and lay department of the hospital, giving the actual amount of work done, the patients treated, number of treatments given, etc. The incorporation of this material into graphs and charts gives the executive and staff a picture of the work of the organization that they can get in no other way. Such graphs are to the administrator what the temperature chart is to the internist. A row of figures is meaningless to most people, but a curved line portrays a picture of activities that no amount of figures or statistical information could show. This is an idea borrowed from industry that the hospital administrator might very well make more use of.

In addition to the regular administrative meeting, the executive should occasionally make trips through the hospital for the purpose of discussing administrative psychiatry with the members of his staff. During these "walks" through the various departments he does not lecture to them but brings up points for free discussion. He will take them into the engineer's department and draw the chief engineer into the discussion. He will have them accompany him to construction work that is going on, in company with the foreman of construction. He will take them into the steward's department and with the steward will discuss the procedures that affect their own particular work. He is not afraid to tell his plans for the future. He gets all the comments that a staff living under these conditions can make. He gets a fund of information which is exceedingly valuable, and he gives his staff the satisfaction of being able to express themselves freely on points that concern them in their work. This is his teaching function.

DELEGATION OF AUTHORITY AND RESPONSIBILITY

An indispensable factor in the successful operation of this kind of management is the ability of the administrator to delegate authority and responsibility. The executive who to a considerable extent cannot relinquish the reins had better never embark on a democratic regime. It is requisite that men in responsible positions make their own decisions. In making them they will turn to anyone who can give them factual material to make the decision sound. These sources of information naturally include the superintendent. "What shall I do?" asks the timid assistant. "What do you think you should do?" replies the executive. In this delegation of authority and responsibility there are two things the assistant must know. He must know exactly what the duties of his position are and how far his authority goes in carrying out these responsibilities.

Many people do not want the responsibility that such a type of organization carries. They prefer to have someone else settle their difficulties with subordinates. Naturally such individuals will not do their best work in a democratic group and should be eliminated as rapidly as possible. It is absolutely essential in this type of organization that every supervising officer stand upon his own feet, make his own decisions, and act with perfect freedom and within the broad limits of the policies of the organization which he represents. He is carrying the responsibility of the reputation of the leader of the group and also the responsibility of the furtherance of his own career. Such responsibilities sometimes make men timid. They are afraid to make such decisions as are necessary in their relationship with subordinates. Such individuals would be better out of the organization. They do not do their best work in this type of administration and the administration invariably suffers from them.

The creative leader will support his assistants in their decisions. He will defend and fight for them, but he will also form some judgments upon the man who gets him into a false position too many times. The staff member who has to be reinforced constantly by the executive is better out of the organization, but there should never be any uncertainty in the mind of any assistant as to whether he will be supported by his superior in any order that he may give to subordinates. The executive who permits the nurse to come to him in protest over a situation which has developed between herself and the supervisor is injuring the morale of his group. By all means see her, but only through appointment arranged by her immediate superior. This is playing fair with both superior and subordinate.

STANDARD PRACTICE

Tradition is the curse of the mental hospital. I do not wish to imply that whatever is old is bad and that which is new is good. But it is impossible for any organization to keep out of a rut unless its practices are being reviewed frequently for the purpose of deciding what is good and what is bad. Groups form habits as do individuals and such habits are more difficult to break than they would be in an individual. The methods of the hospital which have been shown by experience to be good must be known to every member of the group if good results are to be attained. The custom of passing such information along by word of mouth is not good practice. Modifications of standard practice should not be left to the whims of individual staff members. Neither should standard practice be handed out by edict. An administrative problem is to be corrected. The administrator will not be so concerned with the method of correction as he will be with the result of the method.

By standard practice I mean the incorporation into a systematic manual of methods which experience has shown to be the best for handling constantly recurring situations. Such a manual is invaluable for those members of the professional staff who are charged with the responsibility of ward administration. It should cover routine procedures such as legal commitments, letters regarding the condition of patients, accidents, escapes, medical treatment and hospitalization of employees, accidents among personnel, telephone service, routine admission procedure, methods of securing specialized service such as laboratory and clinic facilities, x-ray studies, the routine practice regarding medical and surgical consultation, the transfer of patients from ward to ward, the procedure in case of death, legal routine in case of sudden death, autopsies, staff meetings, preparation of patients' records, deportation proceedings, Board of Health regulations, narcotic laws, diets, statistical material, procedures of patients leaving the hospital, etc. Many other points will occur to the administrator. This standard practice can be built up by the medical staff. Each point should be freely discussed, and after such discussion the chairman of the meeting dictates to the stenographer the exact procedure as agreed to by the staff and in the hearing of the latter, so that any corrections may be made before the matter is put into typewritten form. When all of the routine medical and psychiatric matters in the hospital are covered in this manner, the material is bound in loose-leaf books and a copy given to each member of the staff. The book must be kept alive and up-to-date, otherwise it becomes a mere tradition. The best way to enlist the interest of the staff in keeping the material from becoming obsolete is to appoint a standard practice committee. This should consist of three members of the staff, either three psychiatrists, or a psychiatrist, the director of nursing, and a supervisor, or any other suitable combination. The exact make-up of the committee would depend somewhat upon the questions which would have to be decided upon. Such a committee should meet monthly and bring to the superintendent recommendations for new standard practice or changes that should be made in the existing routine.

In addition to this general standard practice, each department should have such a manual dealing with the details of the work within that department. There should be a standard practice for the admission of new patients, one for the medical and surgical service, one for the psychiatric nursing service, and similar manuals for both professional and lay divisions of the hospital. The administrator who seeks to put down in black and white the actual practices of his hospital will be astonished at the magnitude of the task. But he will be more than gratified by the results in better morale that such a standard practice brings.

My personal experience over a period of twenty-five years is that there is entirely too much uncertainty on the part of the staff members as to what the hospital stands for, what the routine practice is, how far the responsibility of each man goes, and just what authority he has for carrying out these responsibilities. Most of this material is passed on by word of mouth with such interpretations and instructions as the least loyal member of the organization sees fit to insert. The result is a state of uncertainty in the minds of everyone as to what support they will have in their attempts to meet situations.

PROFESSIONAL GROUPS OTHER THAN MEDICAL

Psychiatry is not exclusively a medical problem. In our present state of knowledge the approach to psychiatry must be a coöperative one. We must allow everyone who has a contribution to offer the opportunity to make it. We have not been too ready in the past to see that other disciplines may have a sound approach to the problem of the psychoses. This attitude will be changed by the creative psychiatric administrator. He will see in an open-door policy an opportunity to broaden his field of service. He will realize that the patient will be benefited, that psychiatric education will be the gainer, and that his own hospital will be the better for having these professional groups as a part of his organization. The psychologist, social worker, graduate nurse, sociologist, clergyman, biochemist, anthropologist, and many other representatives of the social and natural sciences are interested in the problem.

It is not good practice to keep them at arm's length. When they are accepted in the organization they immediately become part of the professional staff with the prestige to which their training and ability entitles them. Their effectiveness cannot be realized if they are in the hospital merely on sufferance.

LAY STAFF

Here we reach an important part of this discussion. There has always been a line of demarcation between the layman and the professional. Neither has appreciated what the other was trying to do and each was irritated by the efforts of the other to do an efficient job. If the administrator is to integrate his organization towards a common goal, he must exert every effort to bring these two groups together. The head of the business department is apt to look upon the earnest psychiatrist or the research psychologist with the amused tolerance one has for the child with his toys. He has no objection to the social worker or the chemist being in the hospital as long as they remain quiet and do not bother him. But he has no particular respect for their ability or the work they are doing because he does not understand it. On the other hand, the research worker thinks of the business departments as made up of individuals whose sole purpose in life is to annoy him by refusing to buy the equipment that he needs in his work. He has no understanding or sympathy for the problems of the man who has to guard the financial integrity of the hospital.

The problem of the hospital administrator is to bring these people together towards a common goal. Inasmuch as the institution is a hospital, that goal must be a professional one. Can these two groups with their different training, viewpoint, and ideals be amalgamated into one harmonious whole? Is it possible for the business man, the farm superintendent, the construction foreman, the chief engineer, and the head housekeeper to be convinced that the real purpose of the hospital is to cure patients? Can they be brought to see that the work they are doing is a contribution towards this purpose? Will they come to the point where they will accept professional guidance? It has been my experience that they will through a participating type of democratic organization.

One of the techniques by which the desired result can be accomplished is through the medium of a department head conference. This is a group made up of the superintendent, assistant superintendent, steward, head farmer, chief engineer, superintendent of construction, treasurer, head housekeeper, and superintendent of nurses. The group acts as a council for the superintendent on business matters. A weekly meeting covers the work of the previous week and plans for the current period. Here the committee idea is again utilized freely. The director of nurses needs a utensil sterilizer for the surgical ward. The steward is doubtful about the financial resources permitting it. A committee is appointed to bring in a report the following week as to what must be done and the cost, the final decision to be made then. The administrator knows his people. When the head of the nursing service says she must have a sterilizer, it is a real need. And the department heads, hearing her explanation, know that the equipment is essential to the well-being of the patients. And so it goes, each learning about the problems of the other. At monthly intervals the head occupational therapist meets with the group and reports on the occupational situation. She tells of patients who have improved as a direct result of work in a department. This creates a sense of responsibility for the treatment of patients. Once each month the medical council and department head group meet and discuss finances. The head social worker reports on boarding out patients. The steward gives a talk on the facts about coffee. So it goes on constantly, each group educating the other, each gaining a respect for the ability and accomplishments of the other, and the result is eventually an acceptance of a common purpose and goal.

Through these methods and techniques one eventually arrives at a point where real loyalty exists in the hospital group—not loyalty based on fear but that which comes because of a belief in what the administrator represents, a faith in the plans and policies, and a willingness to follow the leader in carrying them out. It is a loyalty which is engendered by constructive leadership but which cannot come from dictatorship. It seems rather obvious that if the executive wishes to secure loyalty from his subordinates it is essential that he be loyal to them.

If he cannot be loyal to them—and this loyalty must be on the basis of a belief in their abilities, their willingness and desire to follow where he leads them—he is not being fair to himself or to his organization. Loyalty works both ways. The leader has a right to expect the loyalty of those who are being led, but on the other hand those who are led have a right to expect the loyalty of the leader. There is one other point about this matter that should be emphasized. Complete integration is only possible when organization members are not only loyal to the leader but to every other member of the group. By this I mean a mutual respect for the contributions of each other and not merely an emotional liking. This interrelationship between members of the group is so important that every effort should be made to create such a feeling between them. It makes the difference between a thoroughly integrated organization and one whose members are pulling in different directions.

Active leadership is essential in the administration of psychiatric hospitals. Such leadership will demand much from a staff. It will set up an atmosphere of intellectual freedom where each individual may think as he likes but will be tolerant of the opinion of others. The goal of the mental hospital must be psychiatric rather than economic if the institution is to be a real, living, breathing hospital. Every administrative process must be made subservient to that goal and the entire staff must be integrated to that end. The autocratic executive will eventually be superseded by the creative leader. Partnership of executive and personnel is one of the aims of mental hospital management. The administrator achieves this by group planning rather than by authority flowing from the top. Committees and group conferences are important factors in attaining this result. They weld groups and departments into a harmonious whole.

Chapter 4

THE NURSING PROBLEM

THE PROBLEM:

THE mental hospital differs from other organizations in one very important respect. Every administrative act, every system set up, every method used in carrying out the purpose of the institution has a relatively profound effect upon the mental state of the patient. It is unquestionable that the administrative routine of the mental hospital plays a significant and important rôle in the progress of most patients. If this be true, the executive bears a special responsibility in relation to therapy. The harmony which exists between hospital and patient may mean the difference between success and failure of treatment by the individual psychotherapist. If the psychiatrist comes to the patient as the representative of an institution which functions smoothly and with a minimum of friction, the rapport between its representative and the patient becomes stronger and more lasting. On the other hand, if the patient has been constantly irritated by tactless handling, exasperated by petty tyrannies, and annoyed by inflexible rules enforced by poorly informed attendants and improperly trained nurses, he soon develops the idea that his welfare is not the first consideration. In such a situation the psychotherapist starts with a definite handicap which may seriously interfere with his efforts.

Every member of the hospital organization has a responsibility in setting up such a harmonious institution-patient relationship. This is largely the result of those forces, both physical and human, which constantly play upon the patient and regulate his daily life. Of these there is one group that is the most powerful factor of all, the ward nursing personnel. The relationship between patient and attendant may make or break the former. Every mental hospital superintendent can relate instances of ward employees who have patiently and laboriously brought seemingly hopelessly deteriorated patients to normality. By apparently good understanding, through broad human sympathy, and with infinite patience they have led the patient step by step back to the world of reality. And yet these instances have apparently taught us few lessons. More sensitive administrators have given much thought to the color of wards. They have selected the furniture carefully and painstakingly, they have put in flowers and birds, and installed pianos and radios. All has been done to improve the patient's physical environment. But the most important part, the social environment as represented by the ward attendant, has been given much less attention. Beautiful surroundings are a hollow mockery when a small-minded, unintelligent attendant constantly thwarts the patient in his attempts to enjoy them. There is a type of psychological abuse of mental patients which may be much more disastrous than any kind of physical abuse. By this I mean the tactless treatment of the patient by an untrained individual, the refusal of small desires and requests, and the abuse of power that is necessarily conferred upon the individual who is in charge of a ward of mental patients.

If the symptoms of the psychotic individual indicate withdrawal from reality, the problem of the hospital is to create a reality that is sufficiently attractive or compelling to give competition to his dream-like world. Hoskins,[18] in his *Dementia Praecox—A Simplified Formulation,* gives us some hint of the problem. He states:

a. Dementia praecox is an intermittently or continuously persisting dream state...
b. The psychosis results from an intolerable feeling of loss of self-respect. This is due to a feeling of failure of the individual to meet his own personal standards...
c. Dementia praecox is characteristically accompanied by a feeling of isolation.
d. The psychosis serves as a protective reaction.

In an article written by John E. Davis,[19] Senior Physical Director of the Veterans' Administration Facility, entitled, "The Attendant in Mental Re-education," we find the following instructions for attendants in their relationship with psychotic patients:

1. Attempt to create an infectious relationship through genuine, personal, kindly, and understanding interest. Learn 'the art of being human.'
2. Make the patient feel at ease and comfortable. Do not attempt to exact too much from an autistic personality at first. Realize the essential slowness of this adjusting process. The most precious and coveted possession of the patient is his individual personality. Make him feel that his rights are guaranteed.
3. Approach the patient on his own intellectual, perceptive, emotional, volitional, and interest level. Study deterioration grades. While this may appear to be a dogmatic formulation, the therapist will readily recall many cases of failure due to a deficient, excessive, or distorted function of these elements of personality.
4. Explain not only the methods of the proposed therapeutic project, but the reason for it. Emphasize its social co-operative nature, and significance in developing the patient's capacity and affording him well-merited recognition.
5. Attempt to restore the patient's self-respect. Direct efforts against the stigma of a psychosis.
6. Utilize educational approach methods and content by
   a. Placing the patient in active controlled situations.
   b. Grading activities from simple one-response to complex many-response activities.
   c. Utilizing the primary performances of automatic reflex and emotional acts as the first stage and the secondary performances of voluntary acts as the second stage of therapeutic activities.
   d. Providing for progression and graduation in formal recognition to the patient who has advanced to a higher grade.
   e. Emphasizing the re-educational force of suitable motivation. The energy utilized by the patient is but a small part of his potential energy.

But where are we to get the ward personnel to understand, interpret, and apply these rules in terms of nursing technique to the patient? Surely the ward attendant with no more than an eighth grade education who applies for work at a mental hospital because there is no other employment to be obtained cannot do it. He may be filled with the "milk of human kindness," he may have the greatest sympathy for the unfortunate, and he may be inspired by the holiest of motives, but he still falls short of fulfilling the requirements because of his inability to acquire the requisite knowledge to carry out a program of this nature. Can we go on with our present personnel trying to meet a challenge like this? Shall we continue to trust in God that the required number of divinely inspired men and women, capable of carrying on a regime calculated to achieve results in recovered patients, will drop into our laps? Shall we continue to emphasize to our legislative bodies the need for more buildings to house more patients, or shall we begin to stress the great need for thought being given to the quantity and quality of personnel that man these buildings? It is only a rationalization to say that conditions cannot be changed. If we fought for such a principle sufficiently long and hard, it would sooner or later be established. When the human elements in the organization are given the same thoughtful consideration that we give to more material matters, the hospital will more often arrive at the real goal—the cure of patients. We write lengthy and detailed specifications for supplies. Can we not write specifications for our ward caretakers?

William A. White [20] says, "With the ideal of kindliness we had been expecting to accomplish everything. Kindliness alone could never solve the problem." We bring into our wards untrained men and women. If they receive training it is of a most superficial character. Quotas are kept so low that in most cases there is no time to give adequate instruction before the employee is put on a ward, frequently on his own responsibility. Yet few industrial concerns will permit new employees to take over regular duties until they have been trained and instructed. The Bell Telephone Company, for instance, gives a four-week period of instruction before a girl is permitted to go on the switchboard, and even if she has had experience, at least two weeks are considered necessary. Yet central control groups do not see the necessity of allowing sufficient ward personnel to permit proper training for those who are employed to deal with psychotic patients. Without understanding or appreciation of the reasons leading to such conduct, we place them on a ward of filthy, destructive, violent, profane, noisy patients and expect them to preserve their attitude of kindness. And yet it is surprising that many of them are able to do exactly this. There are a considerable number who can preserve their emotional equilibrium and remain humane, even under these conditions. But it is only because of their fundamental decency and not because they have any spark of real understanding of the fundamental situation.

White (*ibid.* p. 80-81) further says, "An attitude on the part of the institution that sees in a restless irritability something to be repressed is not only unintelligent but invites a continuation of the very condition it is trying to do away with and helps by the very repressive measures used to effect this end and to create and continue that patient-institution disharmony upon which it is frequently based. In an institution dominated by the ideal of scientific knowledge, this ideal will so permeate the atmosphere and its effects will be so profound upon the staff, upon the employees, upon all in fact, that there will gradually grow out of such a standpoint a hospital finally and everlastingly free from the shackles of fear and ignorance, a hospital in which the patient will be received with an understanding attitude. And when they are so dealt with, the number of violent outbreaks, serious injury, or resorting to terrorizing and repressing measures will sink to an inconsiderable minimum."

I have been connected with mental hospitals too long not to appreciate the difficulties inherent in this situation. I am thoroughly familiar with the pressure on the administrator to "cover the wards." I am acquainted with the importunities that come from the outside to employ this or that individual regardless of his fitness for ward duty. I am not unmindful of the heartaches and disappointments that come from attempts to inculcate a spirit of understanding into a group of ward attendants. And yet in spite of these difficulties I cannot feel that attempts to change the situation are impossible. Surely something can be done to increase the number and improve the quality of ward personnel.

My suggestion is that we turn to the nursing profession for

a more understanding and better trained service for our patients. This may not be the complete solution of the problem of psychiatric nursing. It is possible that out of attempts to improve the situation a new profession will emerge, the members of which will be specially educated for psychiatric work—a group of individuals with a background combining to some extent that of education and psychiatry. It may very well be that out of this situation will develop the counsellor type of ward leader who will be able, by means of her special training and interest in the work, to organize patients for work and play and in addition carry on some psychotherapy under the guidance of the psychiatrist. But such a profession seems to be in the far distant future. At present I believe we must turn to the graduate nurse for help in solving our problem.

The grading committee of the League of Nursing Education in an admirable report on the nursing situation throughout the United States, *Nursing Schools—Today and Tomorrow*,[21] states that "unemployment in general nursing is not a development of the economic depression. When the Committee started its work in 1926, nursing unemployment was serious. During the prosperity period of 1927, 1928, and 1929, as from 1930 on, nursing has suffered from widespread unemployment. During the past thirty years the population of the United States has increased 62 per cent while the number of trained nurses has increased 2,374 per cent. Approximately 100,000 new nurses have been added to the profession during the past four years (1934). In 1900 there was one trained nurse to every 6,389 people. By 1930 there was one trained nurse to every 416 people." Do not these figures give the mental hospital superintendent food for thought? Would not these gradate nurses be good material for mental hospitals and immensely superior to inexperienced and untrained ward attendants?

The nursing care and treatment of mental patients is a complicated technique. The psychiatric nurse must have more training and experience than the nurse who cares for physically ill patients. Good mental nursing calls for the greatest understanding of human nature, both in illness and in health, an unlimited amount of patience, and particularly the ability to detect and take advantage of every minor psychological change that the patient shows in order that his attitude towards life may be turned into more normal channels. If we are to have more than mere custodial care for our patients we must have individuals who are specially trained to nurse them. Merely filling jobs in a mental hospital results in our not having nurses but guards and keepers.

The idea that *anyone* can work on the wards of a mental hospital must be changed. It is a nursing specialty for which candidates must be properly trained and educated. The nurse who is competent to handle the problems that arise on a ward filled with mental patients and who can make a real contribution to their recovery obtains this competence only as a result of experience and training, built on the proper personality. Not everyone has the requisite poise and temperament that enables one to get along with people who are suffering from mental disorder. Even graduate nurses cannot always understand the psychological differences between these patients unless they have this special training. "Crazy people" are "crazy" to the untrained person, but to the specially educated psychiatric nurse there are as many differences between psychotic patients as there are between so-called normal individuals. Some of the reasons for the use of graduate nurses instead of attendants in mental hospitals seem worth while discussing at somewhat greater length.

Economy of time and money. The graduate nurse comes to us thoroughly trained in the simple nursing techniques that are so essential in any kind of hospital. She can take temperatures, give enemas, and record observations. The many technical procedures that are necessary in nursing the sick properly are understood by her. We do not have to give her training in these fundamentals. The untrained attendant cannot carry out such nursing procedures without a long and expensive educational process.

Specially trained graduate nurses raise the standards of care of patients from the custodial to the nursing level. They have the experience and understanding that enable them to organize patients into recreational, occupational, and ordinary hygiene groups instead of permitting these patients to sit about in idleness, immersed in their abnormal thoughts. The well-trained psychiatric nurse sees that every patient is employed in some way. She seeks constantly to substitute for the brooding thoughts that so engross the patient to the exclusion of everything else, a more healthy and normal outlet that is nearer reality. The ability to administer a ward on such a basis comes only with experience and special training.

The psychiatrically educated nurse makes intelligent observations regarding the symptoms of patients. This gives the physician an opportunity to have the services of a real assistant rather than a mere order-taker, and he is able to do much more for his patients through her rapport. She lives on the ward with them for many hours each day. She knows the significance of a silly grin, a change in attitude, a beginning depressive attack with suicide as a danger. She understands the possibility of accidents that come from the fragile and easily fractured bones of patients who are suffering from certain types of mental disease. She appreciates the necessity of taking precautions to prevent such accidents. Many of the regrettable accidents that have happened to patients in mental hospitals have been due to untrained ward personnel who do not understand the significance of these small psychological changes that come in the lives of our patients.

Graduate nurses are trained in discipline and administration. Ward personnel must have competent nursing leadership. The ward attendant must be directed by an experienced and well-trained nurse who knows mental nursing and what can be done with and for a mental patient. We must have employees who will accept that direction cheerfully and willingly and with a full appreciation of its benefits to the patient. Many people—even graduate nurses—are totally unfitted to work under the rather rigid discipline that prevails in a mental hospital where the relationship between ward employee and patient is so close and important.

There are numerous indications that graduate nurses are turning to psychiatric nursing. This movement will increase if mental hospitals will utilize them. The trend is quite apart from the economic situation. Nursing educators are recognizing the fact that psychiatric experience is necessary to a well-educated nurse, and they are turning to the mental hospital for such training and experience. The substitution of the nurse for the attendant is a progressive move. With her general nursing education, supplemented by special psychiatric instruction, she will become a powerful factor in the psychiatric team.

Organization of Nursing Service.

The traditional organization of the psychiatric hospital nursing service is to have a superintendent of nurses in charge of the nursing school and women's wards. The nursing of men patients is left in charge of a male supervisor who is responsible directly to the superintendent.

This plan of nursing organization is wrong from both the administrative and the humanitarian standpoints. From the first point of view, two heads to any department is not good administrative procedure. Responsibility is divided, rivalry is set up, and the hospital is apt to be divided into male and female camps. It does not make for good integration. From the second point of view, why should there be two standards of nursing care in one hospital? I have known student nurses to graduate from mental hospital training schools without having had any experience on the male wards. The same standard of nursing care should prevail throughout the hospital. The nursing service should be headed by one individual, a director of nursing, and she should be held responsible for the standards of care for both sexes. This is the first step towards psychiatric nursing rather than guard service.

The director of nursing who is capable of assuming this responsibility must be carefully selected as to cultural background, general and special nursing education, ability as an administrator, and general fitness for the task in hand. She must be selected as carefully and conscientiously as one would engage an assistant superintendent or any other high-ranking officer. For her department is one of the most important in the organization.

The social status of the nursing group in the organization of many mental hospitals has been slightly below that of clerks, stenographers, and office assistants. This condition must be completely changed if we are to attract the type of individual who is capable of organizing and managing such a complicated and intricate service as the nursing in a large mental hospital. The head of such a department must be able to gain and maintain the respect of professional and lay department heads, both by her background and experience and by her ability as a nursing administrator. She must be able to meet them on equal terms.

THE DIRECTOR OF NURSING

What should be the qualifications of a director? I offer the following as fulfilling the requirements that I believe necessary for the person who occupies such a responsible position:

1. College training leading to a bachelor's degree. This should give her the general cultural background necessary.
2. A degree from a recognized school of nursing education or graduation from a general hospital school known for the superior quality of its graduates.
3. Experience of at least three years in general hospital administration as head nurse, supervisor, instructor, or superintendent of nurses.
4. Postgraduate course in psychiatric nursing in one of the recognized centers where such education is to be obtained.
5. At least three years' administration experience in a first class psychiatric hospital.
6. Short courses in administration, teaching, and similar branches of nursing would be an asset.

I can hear the comments of some of my colleagues when they read these requirements. "Utopian," says one. "Ridiculous," exclaims another. "Where can we get such people?" But in spite of skepticism, I maintain the position that more radical reforms in the treatment of insane patients have been achieved when the need for them was frankly faced.

Except in unusual instances where individuals have shown special ability, these should be the educational requirements for the head of the nursing service in any mental hospital. But these are not all the qualifications needed. She must be one who is interested in her general professional group. She should be a leader in her nursing organization. She must be sufficiently well known in nursing circles to attract other women of high calibre. It is in this way that we shall secure the best people for our hospitals. It seems needless to say that she must demonstrate her qualities as an organizer and a leader in her department. She must be able to get along well with her superiors, her equals, and her subordinates. She must be a real teacher and stimulator. These are unusual requirements. But the position to be filled is a difficult one.

ASSISTANT DIRECTOR OF NURSING

The qualifications that are given for the director of nursing are equally applicable to one who is to fill this position. She shares the duties and responsibilities of the former and is in direct charge during her absence, and she is the one who should be ready to assume charge if the director leaves. She must be selected with the greatest care and her position in the organization must be consistent with her education and ability. The assistant director should have high nursing ideals, good administrative ability, and a personality that enables her to carry out those democratic principles of organization of which this book is an exponent.

Such nursing executives can and will be found as soon as mental hospital administrators indicate their desire to utilize them. Few have thus far entered the service because the opportunities in psychiatric nursing have not been apparent.

It is not entirely a question of money, fine nurses' homes, or good living conditions. It is rather a matter of spirit, hospital atmosphere, ideals, and above all, an actual nursing policy that is in accord with present-day nursing trends. It is the chance to become creative nursing leaders that will attract them. It is the challenge of psychiatry that appeals. With such nursing leadership every supervisor will be of superior education and training and the total effect will eventually be to have each ward in charge of a competent, well-educated, and psychiatrically trained nurse. When this is accomplished we shall have true psychiatric nursing.

SUPERVISORS

Most organizations have a chief supervisor for each side of the hospital and assistant supervisors for the different services. The chief supervisor is responsible to the director of nursing. The following seem reasonable qualifications necessary for a supervisor:

1. High school graduation.
2. Graduation from an approved training school.
3. Two years' general hospital experience or private duty nursing.
4. At least one year of mental hospital experience as a head nurse or postgraduate student.

Graduates of mental hospital nursing schools should have at least one year of postgraduate experience in an approved general hospital or an equivalent period in private duty nursing.

Supervisors must have administrative ability. They should be able to plan, organize, and act in the capacity of teachers. They should be more than mere order-takers. They are the minor executives of the nursing service and as such they must show leadership qualities.

SPECIAL SUPERVISORS

Working Group. The supervision of the care and treatment of patients working on the grounds, gardens, and fields calls for the services of a special type of supervisor. Here the graduate nurse would be of little value. Such a supervisor must have, in addition to his knowledge of patients and their treatment, an exceptional ability to organize them in groups for work. He or she must be able to direct the attendants who are immediately in charge of patients.

Housekeeping Supervisor. Housekeeping is a specialized activity in the mental hospital. While this work is properly utilized as treatment, the standard and general supervision should be the responsibility of a special supervisor. It is a matter of what the standards should be rather than the methods of attaining them. The ward personnel must devise the means by which good housekeeping is attained, but the supervisor should be the one who decides whether they have met these standards. Such an individual need not be a graduate nurse but she must have had experience in hotel or institution housekeeping and have administrative ability. She should be responsible to the director of nursing.

THE HEAD NURSE

Of all the individuals who make up the personnel of a mental hospital the head nurse is the most important from the point of view of patient care and treatment. She is the one who, more than any other person, has the opportunity to carry out psychiatric therapy. She regulates the life and environment of the patient to his detriment or advantage and she can do more to assist or retard his recovery than anyone else. She should be selected with the greatest care and meet the most rigid requirements. Inasmuch as supervisors are frequently promoted from this group, the same general requirements are appropriate:

1. High school education.
2. Graduation from an approved school of nursing.
3. Experience in general hospital or private duty nursing.
4. Experience of at least one year in a psychiatric hospital as an employee or as a postgraduate student.

The personality traits of the ideal psychiatric nurse are difficult to define. But in general one may say that she should have a considerable degree of emotional stability, patience, a sense of humor, and sincere liking for people. High nursing ideals will develop out of a sincere longing to help them. She must have a strong sense of responsibility and loyalty, both to her patient and to the principles of the organization. Ability to adapt readily to changing conditions and a willingness to accept new methods and techniques are important. She should be neat and of professional appearance and manner, be a good detailist, able to make observations and record them accurately, and above all she must show teaching ability. If she is to be a good ward administrator, teaching patients and subordinates is an important part of her responsibility.

Floor Duty Nurse. This is a classification of the nursing

group that is common to general hospitals but not ordinarily used by the mental institution. The floor duty nurse is comparable to the charge attendant except that she does not have the responsibility of the ward. It is from this group that head nurses are selected, hence the qualifications for the general nurse should be for the most part the same as for the head nurse and supervisor. She is subordinate to the head nurse but above the attendant in rank.

The Attendant. In my advocacy of a mental hospital nursing service built around the graduate nurse rather than the attendant, I am not unmindful of the splendid contribution of many men and women attendants to the recovery of psychotic patients. Every administrator knows countless instances where loyal and understanding attendants have been of great value in the therapeutic program of the hospital. What I am discussing is a principle and not individual cases. There will always be a place for attendants, but it must be a situation for which they are fitted. The leadership cannot be in their hands as has been the case in the past. No longer should we build the nursing service around them. On every male ward there must always be one or more men attendants under the direct supervision of the head nurse. The ward housekeeping would be one of the responsibilities the attendant is competent to take, but always under the supervision of the nurse. The latter would particularly concern herself with actual psychiatric nursing, along with the supervision of attendants.

The problem of the female nurse on the male ward arises, and raises the question of possible violence. Presumably violence to the nurse by male patients would come because of an erotic excitement generated by her presence on the ward. But is it true that such a large proportion of male psychotics are heterosexual? And if they are so completely withdrawn from reality, is the heterosexual urge so powerful that it will cause such a situation? Does not the presence of a woman nurse give a sense of security to the homosexual patient, while the male attendant's presence would constantly threaten his emotional security? After considerable experience I am convinced that the danger of violence for the nurse from the male patient is not only no greater than it would be for the male attendant but on the contrary it is considerably less. I have seen only isolated instances of such behavior, and most of them could have been prevented by a better knowledge of the patient and a deeper psychiatric insight on the part of both psychiatrist and nurse. Careful classification is the answer to the problem. In my opinion there is no ward in the mental hospital that would not be improved by having a carefully selected, well-trained psychiatric nurse in charge. Again it is a question of the application of our psychiatric knowledge to an administrative problem. The settlement of such a question is different from that faced by the industrial executive who is confronted with the necessity of placing his men advantageously. And yet even he makes an effort to study his people and place the round pegs in the round holes.

Many who read this chapter may feel that such an organization as I have outlined is entirely impracticable. Such a viewpoint may be correct if we think only of the present. What has been suggested is an ideal of the kind of nursing organization that we should like, which will perhaps take years to achieve but which I still maintain is practicable. Let us hope that another Dorothea Dix will not be necessary to force us to our duty.

Nursing Administration. It is essential in a mental hospital organization to keep a close check on members of the nursing group in order to know who is outstanding and thus marked for promotion, who should be eliminated from the organization, who should be encouraged, and who should be warned. Here again we turn to the committee system. A personnel committee which decides upon ratings, promotions, and demotions is invaluable in any democratic organization. It is unfair to nurse and attendant and to the director of nursing to require that the latter assume the sole responsibility of making such decisions.

I realize that rating systems have many defects and that they do not always give a true picture of an individual's worth. But, imperfect as such a method may be, it is fairer to all than to depend upon the personal judgment of a single individual. In addition it has the value of indicating to the employee concrete weaknesses and strengths and showing exactly what her immediate superiors think of her.

The following rating scheme has been tried and found workable in a mental hospital nursing service. The method of using it is as follows:

Only head nurses and charge attendants are graded unless promotion is being considered. It would be an improvement if all ward personnel were rated, but lack of time prevents this. The system is so worked that four individuals are graded each week and each supervisor, head nurse, and charge attendant receives a rating at six-month intervals. A work sheet is handed to everyone who has supervision of the activity of each individual to be graded. They have a week in which to make these estimates. Supervisors, assistant supervisors, and physicians are the ones who come most closely in touch with the work of the nurse. In the case of floor duty nurses or attendants where promotion is being considered, the head nurse grades the employee. The personnel committee consists of the superintendent, director of nursing, the senior physician of each service, and the two chief supervisors. The committee meets once a week. All individuals who have graded the working sheet must be present to defend the rating. There are always three estimates, and frequently five, each one being made independently. The superintendent acts as the chairman and records the grades on the permanent sheet. If there is a difference of opinion, the matter is discussed and usually the majority opinion is recorded, but everyone must defend his or her grading and give instances to prove the point. Remarks and comments are entered on the permanent record. After the grading has been completed, the employee is shown the grades she has received and the implications discussed.

Employees are graded under three major divisions, each of which has five subdivisions:

A. *Ward Administration*
  a. Housekeeping
  b. Supervision of Other Employees
  c. Patient Destruction on Ward
  d. Organization of Patients
  e. Records

B. *Interest in Work*
  a. Interest in Patients
  b. Patients' Reaction to Employee
  c. Knowledge about Patients
  d. Professional Attitude
  e. Loyalty to Hospital

C. *General Traits*
  a. Punctuality
  b. Sense of Responsibility
  c. Personal Appearance
  d. Social Relationships
  e. Health

This is the material that is finally recorded on the chart. (See Chart No. I.)

On the actual grading sheet five questions are asked under each subdivision. Each question is scored ½ — 1 — 1½ — 2. A perfect score on the subdivision would be 10. The total possible number of points is 150 and the percentage of efficiency can easily be worked out.

The manual of instruction for the rating scale gives the following points to be noted and graded:

Housekeeping

1. What is the general appearance of her ward or wards?

Every ward gives a distinct impression, either good or bad. Appearance, odors, general condition of furniture, curtains, and pictures should be noted.

2. Are the linen rooms, toilets, and floors clean and orderly?

Orderliness and neatness should be noted as well as cleanliness. A cluttered linen room, a toilet unclean, odoriferous, and with cleaning utensils piled about, should receive a zero rating.

3. Are the patients' rooms clean, neat, and orderly?

Most patients are hoarders and tend to accumulate much useless material. Their rooms should be reasonably neat and orderly. If they are not, the condition indicates that the nurse is not a good housekeeper or that she has no control over the patients.

CHART I.

WORCESTER STATE HOSPITAL

Ward Employees' Rating Sheet

Name____________________ Position____________________

Entered Service____________ Promotion_______ Date____________

Date of Rating																								
Number of Question	1	2	3	4	5	T	1	2	3	4	5	T	1	2	3	4	5	T	1	2	3	4	5	T
WARD ADMINISTRATION																								
Housekeeping																								
Supervision of Other Employees																								
Patient Destruction On Ward																								
Organization of Patients																								
Records																								
INTEREST IN WORK																								
Interest in Patients																								
Patients' Reaction to Employee																								
Knowledge About Patients																								
Professional Attitude																								
Loyalty to Hospital																								
GENERAL TRAITS																								
Punctuality																								
Sense of Responsibility																								
Personal Appearance																								
Social Relationships																								
Health																								
TOTAL RATING																								

Remarks____

4. Has she organized patients and nurses for housekeeping?

Ward organization is a valuable way of estimating her ability as a ward administrator. A definite schedule and system is necessary for efficient administration. Have her explain in detail what the daily procedure is.

5. Has she made suggestions for improvement?

If the employee has made one that is practical or if she has shown some initiative by inaugurating new methods or systems, she should have a good grade on this point. Credit should always be given for initiative.

Supervision of Other Employees

1. Has she the ability to supervise subordinates without friction?

The ability to direct the work of others is an important trait in ward administration. Information on this point may be obtained from observation and constant contact with the ward.

2. Does she command their respect and maintain good discipline?

Discipline is necessary on a ward but it should come from the respect of the subordinate for the superior ability of the head nurse. Do you respect her? If you do, her subordinates probably do also.

3. Is her attitude towards them fair?

Many nurses are not objective in their administrative relationships but use their emotions instead of their intellects. Popularity is usually an indication of laxness; respect implies fair treatment.

4. Does she report to her superiors infractions of the rules?

The head nurse is in a position of authority and responsibility. She must have a certain loyalty to the hospital that impels her to report serious infractions of rules and policies to her superiors. One instance entitles the individual to a perfect score.

5. Does she hold her subordinates to a high standard of performance?

The head nurse or supervisor must be a teacher. She must formulate standards and make her subordinates live up to them. If she cannot do this, she does not deserve a high grade.

Ward Destruction

1. What is her attitude towards patient destruction?

Nurses can decrease destruction by substitution methods. Occupation will accomplish a great deal in this direction. Specific information on this point may be obtained from a weekly destruction report from each ward.

2. Is she waste conscious?

Ward inventories are specific sources of information. Carelessness in the use of supplies would call for a low rating on this point.

3. Is she careful of state property?

A study of the employee's repair requests will aid in scoring this accurately. Nurses who fail to ask for repairs promptly are not very careful of state property.

4. Is she careful of food and supplies?

Requisitions from the ward should be studied. If they show thought and care she should receive a high grade. If they are obviously copied from the previous one, the grade should be low.

5. Has she advanced any ideas to prevent waste?

A nurse who is interested and working for the hospital will be alert to devise new methods of waste control. One suggestion should give her a good rating.

Organization of Patients

1. Does she organize personnel for work and play?

This is an important part of the therapy of mental disorder. The nurse who cannot do this is of little use to the hospital no matter how good she is in other fields. Orderly, systematic work and play projects call for high rating. No organization or interest in this phase of nursing calls for a low grade.

2. Has she an interest in the appearance of patients?

The appearance of her patients, day by day, will give positive information on this point. A good psychiatric nurse will see that patients mend their clothes and sew on buttons. A poor one neglects these matters.

3. Are patients permitted to sit about idle?

Patients must be urged to do things. Idle patients on a ward call for a low rating on this point. A nurse who cannot see the value of occupation is a poor psychiatric nurse.

4. Has she a good organization for the daily routine?

Organization is the soul of hospital psychiatric nursing. Without it, little can be accomplished. Keeping patients busy indicates a good nurse; having a regular schedule of routine indicates a good ward administrator.

5. Does she keep the clothing of patients in good repair?

This is easily graded on the general appearance of her patients. The nurse who is not interested in having the patients mend their own clothes should be given a low rating on this point.

Records

1. Are the ward records up-to-date?

A record is of little value if it is not made promptly after the event occurs. The general contact with the ward will give information to both supervisor and physician on this point.

2. Are the records accurate?

It is important that reports be accurate because statistical information depends upon them. Falsifying records or making them out in advance calls for dismissal from the service. Scoring on this point should be carefully done.

3. Are the ward charts showing patient activities properly kept?

A careful examination of these charts is essential to correct grading. Go over the chart with the nurse, item by item. Analyze the chart and make the score on the basis of this analysis.

4. Do the records show thought in preparation?

Records that give little information are of no value. Inspect observation notes, accident records, daily ward reports. Inaccurate or meager reports count against the employee.

5. Are the records of help in the diagnosis and treatment of patients?

Observation notes made on patients by nurses are of great value to the psychiatrist if they represent actual observation. Perfunctory notes are of no value to anyone.

Interest in Work

1. Does she have a real interest in the problems of patients?

The curse of the mental hospital is frequently the attitude of ward personnel. They are keepers rather than nurses. What is her attitude towards restraint, seclusion, and sedation? Are they her first or last resort?

2. Is she rough physically or vocally with patients?

A loud, harsh, grating voice or a brusque manner deserves a low rating. Any suspicion of abuse should call for dismissal, not rating. The employee who sees a patient treated roughly and does not report it is to be held equally guilty with the one who commits the act.

3. Does she try to get extra things for her patients?

This is a good index of her actual interest in her patients. It indicates that she is human and would deserve a good rating.

4. Does she discipline patients through her understanding?

Discipline must be maintained among patients but it should be done in an understanding way. The ability to do this calls for a high grade.

5. Has she suggested new methods of treatment?

Suggestions should be encouraged. The only way a hospital can progress is by trying new methods. The failure to suggest anything new calls for a zero rating.

Patients' Reaction to Employee

1. Do patients generally like her?

This can be judged from the attitude patients have towards the employee. The experienced supervisor or psychiatrist should be able to evaluate this point without difficulty.

2. Do patients coöperate with her willingly and cheerfully?

The rapport that ward personnel gains with patients is an important factor in their recovery. The nurse who is able to inspire confidence in her patients and who gets their coöperation through this deserves a high rating.

3. Would you be satisfied to have her care for your relative?

This is a point in which the emotions rather than the intellect govern the rating. It is an excellent way of judging the value of a psychiatric nurse.

4. Is she really trying to get patients well?

Some nurses hold a job and others are really trying to help patients recover. It is important to know to which group the employee belongs.

5. What do the relatives of patients think of her?

The psychiatrist and supervisor should make special inquiries on this point. What complaints have been registered against her ward and what commendatory observations?

Knowledge about Patients

1. Does she know the details of care and treatment of patients?

To be a real psychiatric assistant to the psychiatrist, the nurse must be able to keep him fully informed regarding the patient. If she cannot do this, she will be of little value to him.

2. Is she familiar with ward organization?

The first duty of a nurse is to teach employees and patients what the daily schedule of the ward is. She cannot do this unless she knows every detail.

3. Does she know about the behavior of individual patients?

She should have accurate knowledge about each patient. Bowels, menstruation, convulsions are all important for consideration in this connection.

4. Does she know about the visitors of patients?

The ward nurse who is interested in her patients will know something about their visitors and the patients' reaction to them.

5. Are her observations helpful in understanding the patient?

In rating this point it is essential that the one who is grading take into consideration the opportunity the nurse has had for making suggestions. Some psychiatrists resent any suggestion of therapy from a nurse, and she should not be penalized under these conditions.

Professional Attitude

1. Does she maintain a professional attitude towards others?

Is she loud, boisterous, or childish in her behavior? Has she dignity and poise?

2. Is she able to take criticism properly?

She may react by becoming sullen and withdrawn. She may be angry or become paranoid under criticism. Or she may react by trying to improve.

3. Is she a teacher for both employees and patients?

Most worth-while teaching is carried on by precept and example. Is she cheerful, pleasant, and reliable?

4. Is she a worthy representative of the hospital in the community?

The community judges the hospital by its contacts with individuals. Is this employee an asset or a liability in this respect?

5. Is she interested in her professional group?

A nurse who does not belong to a general nursing and alumnae organization has little interest in her profession. She should belong, attend meetings, and take part in the activities.

Loyalty to Hospital

1. Does she represent the hospital properly to new employees?

Does she tell them the good things about the hospital or only the bad points?

2. Is she a complainer?

Some complaints are legitimate but we frequently have employees who can see no good in anything. This is a bad mental attitude.

3. Is she loyal to the organization?

Is she loyal through fear of losing her position or loyal because she believes in the policies and ideals of the hospital?

4. Is she a clock-watcher?

The question to be answered is whether she works willingly and cheerfully in emergencies or does she demand her exact time.

5. Does she have a proper pride in her position?

It is important to know what the motives are that induce the individual to give real service. Pride in one's position is an important point to be scored.

Punctuality

1. Does she get reports in on time?

Careful scoring is essential on this point. Procrastination is a serious defect in a nurse.

2. Does she carry out orders promptly?

Good nursing calls for a high score on this point. It is the essence of psychiatric nursing.

3. Does she ask for extra time off duty?

While the policy of the hospital is one of liberality in this respect, there are individuals who take advantage.

4. Does she try to get others to substitute for her without permission?

All such exchanges of time should come through the supervisor. Employees who make their own arrangements are cheating, and a continual disregard of a rule of this kind should call for discharge rather than a low rating.

5. Is she punctual in coming on duty?

A low score on this point indicates lack of consideration for others.

Sense of Responsibility

1. Does she carry out orders without being reminded?

Treatment orders are given for the good of the patient and if they are not carried out, he suffers. An accurate score on this point is essential for a correct rating.

2. Does she make excuses and give alibis?

Some employees react to mistakes by excuses. Others admit the mistake, make promises to do better, and then forget. Still others improve as a result of mistakes. To which group does she belong?

3. Does she accept responsibility for the acts of her subordinates?

This is an index of her fitness for promotion. The ability to hold subordinates to a high level of accomplishment and to accept the responsiblity for their acts indicates a valuable personality trait.

4. Is she industrious?

Does she work within the limits of her physical capacity or is she frequently found sitting down doing nothing?

5. Does she evade the hospital rules and regulations?

Definite regulations are necessary in a mental hospital. Attempts to evade or break them indicates a bad attitude.

Personal Appearance

1. Is she cleanly in her person and habits?

Personal appearance may be an index of mental orderliness.

2. Does she keep her uniform neat and orderly?

Wearing patched or soiled uniforms, uncombed hair, unbuttoned white coats should call for a low rating.

3. Does she keep her room neat and orderly?

Frequent inspection will give positive information on this point.

4. Is she a good example for the patients?

We cannot expect patients to be neat if nurses do not set an example.

5. Does she have a professional appearance?

Extremes of stature, marked obesity, or slimness are not desirable. Neither extreme beauty nor ugliness should get a high score.

Social Relationships

1. Is she socially acceptable to her fellow-workers?

A certain amount of social popularity indicates personality traits that are valuable.

2. Do her social relationships lead her into difficulties?

Social situations may be responsible for an employee's becoming an administrative problem.

3. What is her standing socially in the nurses' home?

The close contacts in the home may show desirable or undesirable personality traits.

4. Does she have any community relationships?

The friends she has outside the hospital community may indicate character traits.

5. Is her character good?

Mental hospitals have frequently been stigmatized by the action of a few employees.

Health

1. What is her general physical condition?

Consult the clinic record for information on this point.

2. Does she report promptly to the employees' clinic when ill?

Employees frequently say nothing about illness until time to go on duty.

3. What are her personal health habits?

Use of alcohol, late hours, no exercise, etc.

4. Has she been hospitalized many times?

Accurate information on this point is available and should be consulted.

5. What is her attitude towards physical illness in patients?

Any carelessness in this respect should call for a low rating.

The psychological effect of this scheme has been, on the whole, good. It gives the administrator an opportunity to know his nursing group better, it enables the psychiatrist to control the distribution of his nursing assistants, and it indicates to the director of nursing the efficiency of both head nurses and supervisors. Perhaps the most interesting by-product of this grading scheme is the information it reveals about the judgment of each person who is actually doing the grading!

Conferences with Nurses

The hospital administrator cannot know intimately every employee in his organization. He cannot meet each one face to face. And if he could it is doubtful whether he could build up that integration towards a single goal as well as it can be done through department heads. Paternalism is inherent in the organization situation. The "father-son" and "father-daughter" rôles played by administrator and employee cannot be disregarded. It tends to set up barriers that are difficult to break down. And possibly if they were broken down, the situation would suffer. At any rate, each department must have its administrative leaders. These leaders, by their closer association with the administrator, should have the principles and policies of the hospital as an integral part of themselves, since they have assisted in formulating them. These leaders must interpret the aims and objects of the institution to their followers and endeavor to adjust the goals of the members of their group to the objects of the organization as a whole. What has been said about leadership in the chapter on "Building a Staff" is equally true of every department head. Participation in planning nursing policies by supervisors and head nurses will create an enthusiastic group of advocates for those policies. A great deal of this can be accomplished through conferences. The superintendent of nurses who meets her supervisors, male and female, each day to discuss plans and routine work, who has her head nurses in conference at least once each week, and the ward psychiatrist who gets his nurses together at regular intervals for the discussion of patients, will have a degree of coöperation which can never be attained under a boss system. They can discuss details of the work, but they are also able to develop the things for which the hospital stands. Conferences are in general well worth the time consumed. The nursing leader will adopt the same committee plan that the administration uses. The question, for example, of patients' making keys is brought up. Instead of suggesting disciplinary measures, would it not be better to form a committee of head nurses and possibly a physician to study ways and means of correcting the situation and bring in a report. Such a method often results in valuable suggestions. This is participative democracy.

RATIO OF NURSES TO PATIENTS

The usual ratio of ward personnel to patients is misleading. To say that a 1 to 8 ratio is proper is not always true, because such a ratio takes no account of admission rate, class of patients, amount of supervision needed, days off duty, illness, or standards of care. Without taking these things into consideration such a ratio appears to be sufficient, but when they are brought into the equation it is soon discovered that the number is entirely inadequate. Physically ill patients require more care than do patients on open wards. The admission wards must have a greater number of nurses and attendants than quiet, continued-treatment wards. Disturbed wards where close supervision is indicated must have a higher ratio than wards where older patients are cared for. In addition to this there are special duties such as operating rooms, X-ray, physiotherapy, hydrotherapy, etc., all of which tend to lower the number of those who actually care for patients. The attempts made by state control organizations to generalize in this matter and say that all hospitals under their jurisdiction shall have a particular ratio are not based upon common sense. Hospitals differ in their standards and the actual work they are doing. The admission rate is not the same, and the more new patients taken in, the higher the ratio should be. There is a great necessity in the administration of a hospital to vary these ratios from time to time as the work increases or decreases. Many patients would be benefited by special nurses or attendants for short intervals, and if such "specials" will hasten the recovery of the patient they should not be withheld. Arbitrary quotas for ward personnel do not constitute good administrative practice. Salary standardization is proper, but quotas should be flexible and based upon a careful study of the work of the individual hospital, its admission and discharge rate, its necessities, and the demands of the patients at different periods. Flexibility will add to efficiency.

Working Time for Ward Personnel

Eight hours is a sufficiently long period for anyone to spend on a ward with psychotic patients. The wear and tear on the nervous system causes fatigue, which may be manifested by irritability, over-strict discipline, and an unreasonable attitude towards patients. It is impossible for anyone to work ten or twelve hours under the conditions that prevail in the mental hospital and not show evidence of this. This is apart from the question of the actual physical work carried on. Industry has recognized the fact that long hours decrease production, and yet many states are still working ward nurses and attendants ten and even twelve hours. The patient always suffers. In an analysis of accidents, it was found that there were two peaks during the twenty-four hours when the greatest number of accidents occurred. One was in the morning between six and seven o'clock, the other occurred in the afternoon between three and five. The first increase was partly due to the fact that attendants came on duty before breakfast. The irritability caused by hunger was undoubtedly responsible for a certain number of accidents. This is shown by the fact that with a rearrangement of the time for breakfast and the requirement that no one come on duty until he had eaten, the number was significantly lessened. But the afternoon peak still continued and this came partly as a result of the fatigue incident to a ten-hour day on the ward. Even though the time is broken up the fatigue is present.

Administrators have frequently looked askance at the eight-hour day because of the fact that three shifts are used and there is one more opportunity to pass the responsibility for ward events along to someone else. But this can be obviated by making *the ward* the unit of administration and holding every head nurse responsible for her ward twenty-four hours a day. If she has the ward organized and her subordinates are loyal to her and to the hospital, the danger of "passing the buck" is minimized. Unless this form of organization is used the patient is liable to suffer from these frequent changes of personnel. Any therapeutic program such as a habit-training regime must be continuous throughout the twenty-four hours. There can be no break in the regularity of the process. If each individual is responsible for the ward only during her duty period, there will be an attempt to evade such responsibility. But with one nurse responsible for the entire period this should not happen.

A second objection which has been raised by administrators is the fact that two-thirds of the organization is off duty constantly and because of the large number of idle employees in the institution, many administrative problems occur. That this is a fact no one can deny. But sooner or later it will be recognized that it is not necessary for everyone connected with a mental hospital to live on the grounds. When housing construction and maintenance costs are taken into consideration it is doubtful if states are really saving money by housing employees in their institutions. In this day of rapid and convenient transportation, there should be no difficulty about living outside as far as many hospitals are concerned. The advantages of such a plan from the standpoint of comfort to the employees would be many. The isolation of the mental hospital is just as deadly to the employees as it is to the professional staff. They do not live normal lives when they are cramped into over-crowded quarters, as they are in many cases. Those who are married are usually cooped up in one or two small rooms and under such conditions it is impossible to have a family. They cannot have normal community contacts and people who work, eat, and sleep together and who have no social relationships outside of their vocational associations soon become very narrow in their outlook.

As I sum up what I have written about this most important administrative department of the mental hospital, I am moved to re-emphasize certain points. The difference between a hospital and an asylum is psychiatric leadership and nursing care. The solution offered seems to me to be the best one available at this time. What the future will bring forth no one can foretell. But with the available resources we have at present, the graduate nurse seems to be our best hope for improving our service to the patient. The substitution of nurses for attendants will bring about a better type of care, which in turn should lead to a higher discharge rate.

A second point which should be stressed is the desirability

of a single standard of care for both men and women. This can only be accomplished by placing all nursing under one responsible head. This head must be one who has the education and personal characteristics that will enable her to assume a real position of leadership in the institution. She must be able, through her prestige in nursing organizations, to attract well-trained nurses to the hospital.

Finally, more nurses are needed in many of our mental hospitals. The custom of generalizing about ratios of ward personnel which takes no account of admission and discharge rates, the kind of service given to the patient, or the number of essential subsidiary departments carried on, is a mistake. All of these should be considered when ward personnel ratios are being worked out.

Chapter 5

STANDARDS OF CARE

THE foundation of all psychiatric hospital treatment is a high level of "custodial" care. The actual physical, psychological, and social attention while the patient is in the hospital is of the utmost importance.

The organization of the ward service so that it may function with the least friction for the patient and the setting up of orderly and systematic methods by which physical, recreational, and hygienic activities are carried on regularly are all included in this term "custodial" care. The problems which arise out of this are peculiar to the mental hospital. The patients admitted are psychotic. Many of them have withdrawn from reality to the extent that they have no interest in the affairs of the world outside themselves. They tend to bog down into a purely vegetative existence. The routine of the hospital may prevent this tendency if the regime is carefully organized and held to a high standard by the administration. When the patient is received into an atmosphere where he is compelled, through pressure of the group, to hold himself to a reasonably high level of behavior, there is less likelihood of his slipping down into the "back ward" type of individual. This standard must confront him from the day he enters the institution. It cannot be delayed until the deterioration process has already begun. One of the objects of a high level of care is prevention.

Psychotic patients may adjust themselves at different levels:

A. *Social Recovery*. By recovery is meant a social adaptation where the individual is able to return to the community and make a reasonably satisfactory adjustment in his work and social life. There may be residual scars, but at least he is able to control his behavior.

B. *Institutional Social Adjustment*. This is the level of adjustment which we so frequently see. It is commonly known as institutionalization. The patient is intact psychologically but settles down into a routine existence in the hospital, accepting the sheltered environment and the fact that other people will regulate his life for him. He is on an open ward, does useful work in the hospital community, bears some responsibility for that work, and on the whole is a useful member of his small group.

C. *Institutional Adjustment.* This is the type of patient that fills the closed "continued treatment" wards. He is able to get along without friction, works either on the ward or under supervision outside, and gives little trouble to the administration except by his attempts to escape. He has not entirely accepted defeat but is using a primitive type of reaction in trying to change the situation.

D. *Deterioration.* At this level the patient succeeds in completely escaping from reality. He lives entirely in his dream world, neglects his personal appearance, has untidy habits, and sits all day in idleness. He is out of contact with the world about him and attempts to bring him back meet with resistance.

The standards of care which prevail in the hospital are responsible to a considerable extent for the level at which patients adjust. If the ideal of the institution is the discharge of patients, if the professional staff is held to a high level of accountability for such discharges, and if administrative mechanisms are set up to bring patients automatically to the attention of the psychiatrists and compel them to defend continued residence in the institution, the last three groups will not be as large as they are.

Many administrators argue that such patients are of more use to society in the hospital than they would be in the community, trying to make an adjustment. But if the institution is to be really a hospital it cannot be content with merely keeping patients. I have noted that no matter how efficient a patient may be in the work he is doing, when he leaves another is soon trained to take his place.

The fourth group is a definite indictment of our therapeutic standards. These people have been permitted to slump into this condition of deterioration because the routine was not sufficiently insistent and compelling to keep them in reality, even for brief intervals.

Simon [22] lists the dangers to which mental patients are subjected as lack of activity, unfavorable surroundings, and lack of responsibility.

The psychotic trying to escape from the world is brought into a hospital situation where there are no demands made upon his adjustment powers except to eat three times a day and to keep out from under foot. He finds this existence to his liking because it leaves plenty of opportunity for his phantasy life. But when he comes into a situation where reality is constantly pressing on him and where he is compelled to perform those daily acts which make him an acceptable member of the group, he cannot escape from reality. He cultivates better habits.

The unfavorable surroundings may be physical or psychological. The psychotic may find his day-dreams more satisfactory because he is living on a dirty ward or because he dislikes an irritable attendant. But when he finds a pleasant environment constantly surrounding him, kindly but firmly turning him away from his phantasies, he will be encouraged to face reality more readily.

Lack of responsibility is an important factor in deterioration. The sheltered life he leads takes away from the patient the necessity for making any decisions. It is all out of his hands. He may protest against this situation, or he may accept it. The protest may become, in itself, a pleasurable experience. But in too many cases the individual stops protesting and settles down into his own phantasy world, retaining only enough interest in his surroundings to get along in a simple situation.

The problem of the administrator is to organize his institution so that the patient will be under this constant pressure of activity. He must be held to a decent level of behavior. It cannot be the same standard that prevails in society, but it must be sufficiently high to compel the attention of the patient. Discipline, the iron hand in the velvet glove, is one of the best kinds of therapy. But always that discipline must be impersonal. The practice of permitting patients to carry on work in a fantastic way, to wear bizarre clothing, or to give expression to their thoughts and ideas in any unusual manner, is not usually for their best interests. There may be cases which should not be interfered with, but these exceptions should be made only on the basis of a careful psychiatric study. Patients are permitted to get into bad habits because of the indifference, lack of understanding, or laziness of the psychiatrists, nurses, and attendants. I have no hesitation in making the statement that a well thought out and properly supervised plan of ward activities will do as much to prevent the accumulation of deteriorated patients on the "back wards" as any single factor in the hospital.

Again the question of personnel arises. The success or failure of any plan of treatment is entirely dependent upon the sympathy, coöperation, and enthusiasm of psychiatrists, supervisors, and ward employees. It requires intelligence, understanding, and long experience and training to appreciate the reasons underlying such a plan. An incident which occurred in a mental hospital aptly illustrates this point. Walking on the ground, I came across a group of deteriorated male patients sitting in idleness while two attendants sat at a distance, keeping an eye on their charges but gossiping and talking with each other. They were watching the patients. They had taken the group out of doors because they had been ordered to and not because they believed that they could accomplish anything. I aroused the attendants from their apathy and set them to work, organizing the patients to carry wood from one pile to another. The task was soon completed and everyone was ready to slump down again. In order to continue the occupation, the attendants were instructed to have the wood carried to another place. It was explained to them that this activity was necessary to prevent the patients from slipping back into their imaginary world. The procedure was repeated several times. It may not have been well planned occupational therapy, but at least it was activity.

That evening one of the attendants came to the office and tendered his resignation. The supervisor, in trying to find the reason for his decision, finally elicited the story about the superintendent having the patients carry the wood. His comment upon the proceeding was, "I won't work in a place where even the superintendent is crazy." Explanations were useless and passed over his head. The patients were crazy and there was nothing to be done about it. Anyone who attempted to do anything was in the same class. What can the administrator do with attendants like this? Custodial care, like everything else in the hospital, can be no better than the abilities of the supervisory and ward personnel which carries it out.

There is the view that some attendants take that it is easier to do a thing than to teach the patient to do it. Ward housekeeping is an end in itself and not a factor in the treatment of sick people. He washes the walls because he is compelled to keep his ward clean, not because he can see in this occupation a way to draw his patients back to reality. In such ways, and in many others, the question of custodial care is intimately bound up in the matter of number and quality of ward personnel.

The institution of a system of care that is calculated to prevent the patient from deteriorating into an apathetic, indifferent individual must begin the moment he enters the hospital. The inculcation of new habits of behavior and thought should be the first consideration, and while he should be received into an atmosphere of kindliness and understanding, the rules of ordinary good conduct must be scrupulously observed.

HABIT TRAINING

It seems obvious that all wards of a mental hospital should have a regime that might be classified as habit training. But the more intensive form is particularly applicable to wards where deteriorated patients reside. There are two problems which confront the administrator. One is prevention. An intensive concentration of effort on the newly-admitted patient will reduce the number of so-called "chronic patients." But until this reduction can actually come about, the problem of what to do with the group we already have is ever before us. For this deteriorated group a ward program of habit training is particularly applicable. At the outset it should be emphasized that habit training performs no miracles. It is not specific for any psychosis. It is not an easy matter to administer a ward on this basis. But if it is enthusiastically followed by physicians and nurses, it will sooner or later transform a hospital. It changes the untidy, disheveled patient into a fairly presentable individual. It lessens the amount of soiled linen sent to the laundry. It cuts down the most repulsive kind of work the ward attendants must do.

But in spite of the advantages and results of a system of habit training, it is exceedingly difficult to get nurses and attendants to carry out such a program faithfully and conscientiously. It is not hard to understand why this should be so, since it involves more work at first for the ward personnel. If the thoughtful administrator goes into the problem thoroughly, he cannot quite escape the conclusion that it is in part the fault of the psychiatrist. The ward employees have not been instructed in the reasons underlying habit training and the results to be obtained. Neither are they held to a high standard of performance. It has seemed to me that there is an unexpressed conviction in the minds of hospital psychiatrists that deteriorated patients cannot be changed. Staff physicians are too ready to accept the fact that the whole problem is a hopeless one.

There are certain principles governing habit training which must be kept in mind if it is to succeed.

1. It cannot be carried on by either psychiatrist or head nurse alone. It is not a one-person job but is the responsibility of everyone who comes in contact with the patient during the entire twenty-four hours. Each must scrupulously carry out the program. There can be no deviation due to the change from one nurse to another. If there are attendants on a ward who cannot or will not understand or who are skeptical as to results, the sooner they are eliminated the better. With them in the team, habit training will fail. Participation on the part of everyone is the first requisite for success.

2. When a routine is established, no change can be permitted for even a day. To do a thing today and forget it tomorrow is disastrous. To carry it out at a different time each day is equally bad. If a patient is to be toileted at 9:15 she must always be taken at that time. A variation of even ten minutes may affect the results.

3. Positive suggestion must take the place of more subtle methods with deteriorated patients. "Button your dress"—"Lace your shoes"—"Comb your hair" are distinct commands which will elicit a response from patients when a less positive

reminder will make no impression. The latter does not cross the threshold of consciousness. This threshold is so high that an extraordinary stimulus must be used. This does not mean that loud and boisterous yelling will bring results. But a firm, decisive voice and manner will cut through the indifference of the patient when a less emphatic tone will not. And here is where the careful and thorough education of the nurse is important. Unless she is well instructed in the psychological principles involved, she may interpret this to mean that a rough and domineering manner is the desirable thing.

Habit training should cover the following aspects:

1. Personal Habits
   a. Intestinal tract
   b. Urinary tract
   c. Care of person
   d. Habits of eating
   e. Personal appearance
2. Physical Exercise
3. Recreation
4. Social Relations.

Intestinal Tract. The matter of bowel incontinence can be corrected by taking the patient to the toilet at the same time each day and leaving him there for fifteen minutes. It may be necessary to do this three times a day. If the incontinence persists after a trial of at least two weeks, a daily enema should be given for three days, followed by a rest of three days. The enema schedule should then be resumed for three days and another rest period of the same length should follow. The enema must always be given at the same time, and after it is completed the patient is placed on the toilet for fifteen minutes. During the three days of rest the toileting must be carried out at the same time the enema would be given. The time factor is an important part of the process. Habit formation is possible for the intestinal tract as well as for other parts of the body.

There are patients in whom enema treatment would be contra-indicated. Physical conditions such as hemorrhoids would preclude its use. There is the patient in whom the enema used in this manner creates an erotic satisfaction. The use of it must always be prescribed by the psychiatrist, and he should be able to exclude from the group such exceptional patients.

Urinary System. Urinary incontinence is somewhat more complicated. Preliminary to any attempt to institute a regime to correct urinary incontinence, a careful survey must be made of the ward to ascertain which patients need correction. This survey should include the following points: (1) Who are the patients that habitually soil themselves or their bed clothing? Most of the untidiness on any ward is caused by a small group of patients, and the intensive work must be done on this group. Therefore it is important to know who these patients are. (2) The time of the incontinence is important. Some patients are nocturnal enuretics; others soil themselves many times, both day and night. Therefore the number of times a day that the patient soils himself is most important.

After the names of the patients and the number of times each soils himself are known, a list should be compiled. A wall board for the use of ward personnel, with spaces for names, is a valuable adjunct to the system. The board should be sufficiently large to have a column for each two hours of the day. It will be found that certain patients will have to be toileted every two hours, both day and night. For those patients who persistently soil themselves this is excellent therapy, and often extraordinary results are attained. Other groups will have to be toileted every four hours, every six hours, etc. It is only in this way that the urinary habits of an entire ward can be changed. But like every other habit-training measure, it requires faithful attention and unremitting vigilance. It can accomplish no more than the people who carry it on will permit.

CARE OF PERSON

The only way by which personal neatness and care of the person can be attained is by quiet, patient persistence. No relaxation should be permitted. Success comes only from eternal watchfulness. What has been said of the other divisions of habit training is equally true of teaching patients to care properly for themselves. There can be no change of routine, either in time or procedure. Care of the person naturally includes the following points:

1. Washing Hands and Face
2. Combing Hair and Brushing Teeth
3. General Bathing
4. Cleaning and Trimming Nails
5. Care of Toe Nails.

GENERAL CARE:

Washing Hands and Face. Every patient in the hospital should be required to wash hands and face and brush the hair three times daily. This personal care is so habitual with all people in our culture that it seems superfluous to even mention it. This may seem to be a trivial matter to which to give much time and thought, but cleanliness would never be the rule unless it were rigidly enforced. The practical difficulties of actually carrying out such a standard deserve much consideration from the administrator. What are the facilities for actually accomplishing this task on a ward of fifty patients? What does it mean in expenditure of time and money? Let us examine the matter in detail. On most wards there are insufficient wash bowls to keep up such a standard. An average length of time necessary for each person to wash face and hands and comb the hair would be ten minutes. Rarely are more than five lavatories installed on a ward. Therefore, with fifty patients and facilities for five at a time, it would take one hour and forty minutes three times daily to carry out this simple function. And if we add five minutes for brushing the teeth once daily, we take up an additional fifty minutes.

This means that if patients have breakfast at 7:00 A.M. some of them must arise at 4:30 in order to make their morning toilet. If the procedure is to be a real habit-training device, every patient must be checked. Many wards have more than fifty patients. If it is done three times daily, under supervision, it consumes approximately five hours of the day for one nurse.

There are still more difficulties to be considered. No one would disagree that with such a standard of cleanliness, the minimum requirement for each patient would be one clean towel daily. Most mental hospitals have a population of at least 2,000 patients. This means that 2,000 towels would have to be issued daily. If the laundry has a linen exchange, good practice would call for a four-point system. That means four towels for each patient. The patient has one, a soiled towel is on the way to the laundry, a clean towel is on the way to the wards, and a clean towel is in the laundry. Therefore, in a 2,000-bed hospital, 8,000 hand towels would have to be in circulation continuously to maintain an ordinarily decent standard of cleanliness.

But this is not all. The soap represents a necessary item of expense. If two-ounce cakes are used, one bar will last six days. This means that 2,000 cakes of soap must be distributed every six days. This amounts to approximately 1,250 pounds of soap per month. If liquid soap is used, the cost is even greater. Therefore, the organization of this simple procedure cannot be left entirely to the ward nurses. They must have the facilities to carry out such a program, which I believe to be therapeutic. It draws the patients back to reality and compels them to have an interest in their personal appearance. It seems obvious that we should build our lavatory rooms and estimate our appropriations on the basis of this need. I have not mentioned waste and replacements, lest the matter get even more complicated than it already is.

Oral Hygiene

The mental hospital employs dentists and hygienists to give care to the teeth of patients. What a needless expenditure of money, if no organized effort is made to carry out the ordinary rules of dental hygiene. Our dental colleagues will agree that a minimum of brushing the teeth once daily is a requirement for dental health. Again we analyze what this means in time and supplies for 2,000 patients. With the same equipment and the same number of patients, we find that the time consumed is fifty minutes each day. Of course in this process the group can be divided into three parts, one brushing the teeth in the morning, one at noon, and the third in the evening. Or the entire group may be required to brush the teeth in the evening before retiring.

The matter of supplies must be considered. A brush such as is used by mental hospitals will last about three months. This means that every patient will use four toothbrushes each year, or a total of 8,000 brushes in a 2,000-bed hospital. Most hospitals prepare a tooth powder which is relatively cheap. One ounce will last approximately a week. This means a weekly distribution of 125 pounds.

BATHING

The question of bathing is an important one. Most mental patients are ambulatory and frequent bathing is an absolute necessity. Dirty clothing and unwashed bodies are responsible for the characteristic odor that was once known as "hospital odor." Here again the question of bathing facilities comes into the matter. There is the old argument between those who advocate tub bathing, and those who believe in showers. The wide use of shower-baths in the general community has given a social approval that makes them acceptable to the mental hospital. The difference of opinion now centers around ward bathing vs. central bathing. On the whole, central bathing seems the more reasonable. While such an arrangement may not be ideal, it is efficient and gives a control to the administrator that he cannot get when each ward has its own bathing facilities. Responsibility is fixed, proper inspections for bruises and skin disease can be made, and records can be kept. The principal objections to central bathing are psychological ones. The opponents maintain that it offends modest patients and in some cases actually causes psychic traumata. This is a perfectly sound objection and would win the argument if it were not true that ward bathing is open to the same objection. There is even less privacy in the ward bathroom than there is in the properly arranged central bathhouse. In a recently completed central bathing suite for women, the matter of exposure is taken care of by having proper dressing and undressing booths. Each patient is given a Turkish towel, sufficiently large to cover the front and back to the knees and with a slit, like a poncho, for the head to go through. This is worn when the patient goes from the booth to the shower stall. It is then taken off and hung across the front of the stall to form a curtain. It is again worn when passing back to the dressing booth. In a properly organized central bath suite, with at least twenty-five showers and fifty dressing booths, every patient can be bathed at least three times per week, and those who work in hospital industries bathed daily. This should be the minimum standard for any mental hospital.

But as in all other processes, there are practical difficulties in the matter of time and money. The shortest period that is consumed in giving a bath, including the undressing process, is twenty minutes. This would not include the trip to and from the wards. With a central suite of twenty-five dressing rooms and an equal number of showers, it would mean that twenty-five patients could be bathed every twenty minutes, or seventy-five per hour. In a population of 2,000, at least 400 are either feeble or in bed. This means that with a suite for men and one for women, one-half of the patients would be bathed daily. This would require eight hours of continuous bathing. Every patient should have a clean Turkish towel for each bath. This would necessitate 1,000 bath towels daily, and if the four-point system were used, 4,000 would be needed. The matter of soap is also a consideration. A two-ounce cake of soap will last a week. This would mean 2,000 cakes per week, or 250 pounds of soap.

In addition to the better standard of cleanliness, frequent shower bathing has a therapeutic effect when properly managed. The bath should start with a temperature of 100° to 105° for its cleansing properties. With water at this temperature the patient should be well soaped. A hot shower is a cerebral excitant and should not be prolonged more than five minutes. It is followed by a shower with the temperature at 97° for a period of ten minutes. With the water at neutral temperature, the shower causes immediate contraction of the cerebral vessels and produces a calming effect on the reflexes. Its effects are essentially the same as those of the neutral immersion bath but are more quickly attained. (Kellogg.[23]) There is in shower bathing an actual hydrotherapeutic effect.

Finger- and Toe-nail Hygiene

Any mental hospital would find it worth while to attach a chiropodist to its staff. The foot troubles of patients are multitudinous. Corns, bunions, and callosities are so frequent as to be commonplace. Careless attendants are frequently responsible for these conditions by their inattention to the footwear of patients. The feet should have an inspection at least once weekly and the nails should be trimmed once in two weeks. A full-time chiropodist will find much to do in the mental hospital. That sore feet, ill-fitting shoes, painful corns, and bunions have a psychological effect on the individual no one can deny. This may not be specific but only irritability and depression due to the pain. The knowledge that the hospital takes no steps to make him comfortable is a fact of some significance.

PERSONAL HYGIENE

Shaving. Here is one of the problems of custodial care that is most difficult to solve, and yet nothing is more depressing than to see patients unshaven and shaggy about the head. The method used by many hospitals is to place barber equipment on each ward and have the shaving done either by a professional barber or the ward attendants. Neither of these methods is satisfactory.

When the work is done by a barber, the chair is brought out on the ward. A patient lathers, the barber shaves, and the patient is sent to a lavatory to wash his face. While there, he usually sticks pieces of toilet paper on the cuts. When the attendants do the shaving there are plenty of these to cover up. Such barber work cannot help but affect the attitude of a patient towards the hospital. I have long advocated the establishment of one or two central shops with modern equipment and of sufficient capacity to shave every male patient at least three times weekly. This is a bare minimum. Patients on open wards should have their own shop where they can be shaved every day. In an open ward shop, about 25 per cent of the patients can shave themselves under the supervision of the barber. They can use safety razors, and in my experience never has an accident occurred. When such shops are in operation, responsibility for the quality of the work can be fixed. Every patient is entitled to proper lathering, a clean, careful shave, a hot towel, a tonic on the face, and talcum powder. If the skin is broken, a styptic stick should be used. I know of no more important factor in maintaining the morale of the patients in a mental hospital than the proper kind of shave in a well-equipped barber shop. It has the same psychological effect as a beauty parlor has on the women patients.

Every patient in the hospital, both men and women, is entitled to a proper haircut every two weeks, not the bizarre "pineapple" type that we see so frequently but a becoming cut which will improve the appearance.

The following standard practice is framed and hung on the wall of the barber shops in a mental hospital, and the regulations are strictly enforced:

STANDARD PRACTICE FOR BARBER SHOPS

The following procedures must be carried out with every patient who is shaved in this shop:

1. Barbers shall use the prescribed towels for the protection of clothing.

2. The patient must be carefully lathered, using soap powder and a clean brush. Lather must be thoroughly rubbed in.

3. Use the safety razor with a sharp blade. Shaving must be done carefully and thoroughly.

4. Any scratches shall have an application of the styptic stick before towels are applied.

5. After shaving a hot towel must be applied to the face.

6. Follow the towel by an application of face lotion, carefully massaging and drying the face.

7. Complete the operation by applying talcum powder.

No deviation from this schedule will be permitted in any case. Whiskers must not be shaved off without permission of the assistant superintendent.

(signed) *Superintendent.*

What are the administrative difficulties in carrying out such a standard? If 35 per cent of the male patients are on open wards and are shaved daily and the remaining 65 per cent are shaved three times a week and all have a haircut once each month, it will require more barbers than are usually allowed in mental hospitals by governing boards. Allowing fifteen minutes for each shave, it would require fifteen barbers working eight hours a day and six days a week to keep 1,000 male patients in decent condition. One barber would do nothing but cut hair. Of course these barbers need not all be employees. Frequently patients can be trained to do excellent work.

WOMEN'S HAIR-DRESSING DIVISION

As far as my reading can give me the information, the first establishment of this kind to be put into a mental hospital was at the Kankakee State Hospital, Kankakee, Illinois. Now most psychiatric institutions have well-equipped hair-dressing rooms, where the standard procedures are carried out by trained beauticians. I know of no factor in the women's side of a mental hospital that has as much value for morale building as this division. The work done there assists in keeping up the self-respect of the patient, the ministrations are soothing and sedative, and the entire effect is beneficial. In this day of bobbed hair for women it is necessary to have a barber for the women's wards. This raises the same question about the number of barbers which has been discussed in relation to the barber shop. The problem, however, is less acute than on the men's side. If 25 per cent of the women have bobbed hair, one barber working an eight-hour day can keep the hair trimmed once in three weeks. This is a good standard.

PHYSICAL EXERCISE

Walking Out-of-Doors. Every patient in the mental hospital should be given the opportunity to walk in the open air at least one hour each day in good weather. The only exception to this rule would be those who have physical disabilities that prevent walking. This rule is important both from the standpoint of health and for psychological reasons. A patient who is walking out-of-doors is assailed by the sights and sounds of nature, which may result in drawing him out into reality for at least a part of the time that he is out. But there are certain traditions that have been built up about even this simple procedure. I know of nothing that is more depressing than the sight of a long line of apathetic patients, shuffling along two by two with uniformed attendants. This is psychological abuse of the worst kind. Think of the humiliation and psychic trauma that a sensitive paranoid patient undergoes in an experience of this kind. The benefit from the exercise in the open air is nullified by the psychological damage. Patients should be taken out in groups of not more than a dozen patients, and the entire arrangement should be as informal and normal as possible.

If there are insufficient attendants to give the proper kind of attention, an exercise yard might be useful. I know many psychiatrists will read this with horror. Yet we must be practical. Such a yard, surrounded by a fence concealed with vines, can be made very attractive. But even here there must be organized activity. To turn a hundred patients into such a yard and permit them to mill about aimlessly is poor therapy. There must be occupation, games, organized play. Playground apparatus in the shape of swings and teeter-boards should be built and installed. This would be an excellent place to carry on flower projects or even gardening. Such out-of-door exercise must be a mental stimulation as well as a physical one if it is to be of any psychiatric value.

Marching on the Ward. If the weather is inclement, ward marching should be carried on for fifteen-minute periods twice a day. All the windows should be raised in order to air the ward, and to the brisk music of a phonograph the patients should be marched up and down the ward as rapidly as they will move for fifteen minutes—again a return to reality.

Calisthenics

Mild calisthenics are an essential part of ward therapy for both men and women. At some period of the day all patients should be lined up on the ward and put through a series of exercises that will benefit them physically and stimulate them mentally.

At this point I wish to make one thing clear. All of these procedures should be carried out as a responsibility of the nurse. They are all involved in psychiatric nursing. Playground and physical instructors could be utilized by the hospital to instruct the nurses and attendants, but in my opinion the latter are the ones who should deal with the patients. All of these measures act to keep patients in touch with reality, and in an ideal hospital situation most of the patients would be kept busy during a large part of their waking hours. In general, physical or mental isolation is bad for the psychotic.

RECREATION

Dances are traditional in the mental hospital. They have been a part of its recreational program since hospitals were first built. But there is a question as to whether these social events have been utilized to the best advantage for a maximum of therapeutic efficiency. The monotonous repetition of the weekly dance held on the same night, the lack of proper selection in the patients attending, the unvarying program carried out, the separation of the sexes, the mediocre music of the average hospital orchestra, and the stiff, unbending, institutional character of the function are not calculated to secure the best psychic therapy. It is rare to hear laughter and to see happy, smiling faces at a mental hospital dance. It is true that psychotic patients have to some extent lost their ability to have social relationships, but something can be done to stimulate a more normal reaction in these dances. That dancing has a stimulating effect no one can deny. That it is a pleasurable experience is equally true. The rhythm of the music, the physical activity, and the contagion of the group all make the dance a particularly valuable therapeutic weapon. But the method of utilizing it needs to be changed.

Weekly dances are too frequent. It is the unexpected that stimulates even the psychotic. Dances held at irregular times once or twice monthly would be more valuable than a monotonous regularity which soon becomes routine and automatic. A better classification of patients attending should be attempted. It is a harrowing experience for the newly-admitted patient to attend this social function and witness the eccentric dancing, bizarre actions, and grotesque costumes of more deteriorated patients. That these latter individuals need the dance is true, but the two groups should not be mixed. It would be better to have two dance functions and graduate a patient from one to the other as a reward for learning to dance properly, adopting a more normal standard of conduct, and developing some pride in personal appearance.

The dance program must be arranged with a view to stimulating the interests of the patient. Special events, novelty numbers, spotlight dances, with an occasional exhibition, would make them more attractive. Prizes for these special events are always stimulating. Instead of the indifferent supervision of a group of attendants who have no interest in the matter except to watch the patients, there should be an alert, vivacious hostess with several carefully selected nurses and attendants to introduce patients to each other, urge the unwilling ones, gently restrain those who are unstable, and keep the function at a fairly good tempo. All of the social amenities should be scrupulously observed. Patients of both sexes must be encouraged to mingle with each other. I do not think that the dangers frequently pointed out need serious consideration. The mental hospital patient leads a strongly homosexual existence, and social functions such as the dance can compensate for this at least to some extent.

The music should be the best that can be procured. Music is a part of the value of the dance. The livelier and better rhythm it has, the more stimulation there is for the patient. The whole function should be a more normal one than it usually is, if it is to be of any great value as a therapeutic measure.

Religious Service

I do not believe that the religious needs of the patients of a mental hospital are best served by the usual custom of inviting local ministers to come to the institution one day each week to hold services. The work of a chaplain in any faith is best carried on with a background of special training and experience. This statement is based upon the fact that every human being has some kind of religious interest, either positive or negative. If this be so, that interest or lack of interest may be one of the avenues through which the patient may be drawn back to reality. I hasten to explain that I do not mean proselytizing the patient or attempting to get him to embrace any particular religious faith or any religion at all. The clergyman has a status with the patient that is different from that of the nurse or psychiatrist, and he can be utilized as a member of the psychiatric team. Under the direction of the psychiatrist and working through his own particular approach, he assists the patient to solve his problems. Church services in mental hospitals, unless conducted by an understanding and well-trained clergyman who has had experience with psychotic patients, can be no more than a mere form. This is particularly true of the Protestant service. The employment of full-time chaplains in mental hospitals would be extremely beneficial for the patients. I would not advocate their living on the grounds, but I believe if the hospital could be their sole responsibility or at least their main responsibility and if they were properly trained and had good experience, they would serve a very useful purpose.

Community Singing

This is a type of recreational activity which is exceedingly valuable in enlisting the interest of the patients and drawing them into reality. To get a large group of patients together in a hall and have them sing under the leadership of a magnetic, inspiring song-leader is one of the finest kinds of therapeutic recreational activities that the mental hospital can have. The contagion of the group, the desire on the part of most human beings to sing, the rhythm required, and the group effort that is involved, all make this particular recreational measure of considerable therapeutic value.

Social Relations

Here we again turn back to the ward and to the responsibility of the ward nurse and attendant. At certain hours of the day every ward should indulge in games of various kinds, group singing, group reading, guessing contests, old-fashioned spelling bees, parties, and similar social activities. The number and variety of these activities are only limited by the ingenuity of the nurses and supervisors in arranging them. Social affairs should be planned between wards, one ward entertaining the other. The patients on a male ward might very well entertain the patients on one of the women's wards. I realize the implication of all this, but again it is entirely a matter of supervision. The rigid homosexual social existence of mental patients does incalculable damage to some. It should again be pointed out that all of these activities of a diversional and recreational character should be under the general supervision of the psychiatrist. If they are to serve as a therapeutic weapon, he should know their possibilities and something about the techniques of using them.

Many administrators will find the ward chart of advantage in keeping a record of the number of patients who are participating in the various divisions of custodial care on the different wards. The number of patients participating under each heading is entered by the nurse at the end of the day, and with careful supervision and frequent checking by supervisors and psychiatrists, such records will be found to be of inestimable value in evaluating the work of the nurse in charge. A high standard of general care in the mental hospital is the backbone of all therapy. The work of specialized individuals must be over and above this general care. The entire organization of the hospital should be built around such care and everything be made subservient to it.

DESTRUCTION

Destruction by deteriorated patients is one of the costly economic leaks in the mental hospital. Whether it should be as high as it is in many institutions is a matter for argument. Whether it can be reduced or is a necessary thing is problematical. The amount of destruction is, in my opinion, in direct proportion to the interest of the head nurse and ward psychiatrist in the matter. We may devise all kinds of restrictive measures, indestructible mattresses, sheets that cannot be torn, strong dresses, and the many other devices that have been tried, but none of them will accomplish what an ingenious, interested, and understanding head nurse and ward psychiatrist can do through the use of occupation, recreation, and general ward activity. If they have an attitude of desiring to know what the behavior of the patient means and if attempts are made to get at the reason for destruction, success will attend such efforts. A substitution of some other activity, the utilization of some bit of history in turning the activities of the patient into socially acceptable channels, a study of the surroundings of the individual may reveal the reason for such behavior. The first step in meeting the problem of destruction is to recognize that there is a problem. The second step in the solution will be the accumulation of data bearing on the matter. Who are the patients that habitually destroy clothing? A classification of the articles each destroys may furnish a clue to the solution. A study of the group which causes most of the destruction, taking note of sex, psychosis, length of time in hospital, and particularly ward relationships, should be undertaken. In the latter the influence of suggestion works both ways, and other patients, nurses, and attendants should be studied. Even psychiatrists themselves may have an influence in the matter. Then the study of the individual patient, his hallucinations, delusions, paranoid reactions, resentments, and other emotional drives and urges is important. A patient may break glass because he wishes to escape, or because he hears voices outside calling to him or hears auditory hallucinations inside that tell him to behave in this way. He may be trying to escape from these voices. He may break the glass as an act of resentment against the hospital or some member of the organization. To attack this problem of destruction in a constructive way, one must be a psychiatric detective, observing the behavior closely for indications of clues leading to motives and making deductions from the evidence that is obtainable. Every patient is a special case. Careful records dealing with this matter are essential if any solution is to be found, and one of the problems of the administrator is to make the entire personnel of the wards conscious of the situation. To accept destruction as an act of God and do nothing about it is to see it mount higher and higher until the cost is appalling. It is a matter of psychiatry and psychiatric nursing.

One way of bringing the matter constantly to the attention of the nursing group is to keep a graphic chart which shows in actual cost the amount of destruction each week. This is placed in a conspicuous place where all employees may see it. An occasional exhibit of destroyed articles may bring the fact to their attention in a dramatic way. But they must become waste-conscious before any change in the situation can be made.

MECHANICAL RESTRAINT

The argument about restraint which has been carried on for so many years is purely an academic discussion. Neither restraint nor non-restraint solves any problem. Like many other factors in the mental hospital, it was the abuse and not the use of restraint that led to its complete abolition. That this was proper no one can deny. Mechanical restraint is practically never indicated in a mental hospital for psychiatric reasons. It is the lazy way of handling these problems. But to substitute other equally lazy ways of meeting the situation does not get us anywhere. Anyone can tie a patient up—it requires no special knowledge or training to do this. But to carefully study a patient, to understand why his behavior is what it is, and then devise ways and means of directing the energy into a socially acceptable form, is psychiatry and psychiatric nursing. A rigid and carefully supervised routine of ward activity will definitely cut down the need for restraint.

HYDROTHERAPY

It is not possible to enter into any exhaustive discussion of this important method of treatment, but the use of the wet-sheet pack has become so involved with the idea of restraint that it should be mentioned. There is no more valuable way of inducing sedation in the unstable and excited patient than a properly applied wet-sheet pack. But here again we see the abuse of an excellent therapeutic procedure leading to its disrepute. It is perfectly true that the application of a wet-sheet pack means restraint for the patient, but it has a decided physiological effect that causes sedation. Packs have been used indiscriminately by ward psychiatrists to restrain patients, and attendants have threatened them with packs to induce good behavior. It has been the bogey of the disturbed ward, until patients fear it and are made more excitable through apprehension. Packs are ordered without knowing whether this is the form of treatment suitable for the particular case.

The use of the wet pack in properly selected cases and with a full understanding of the principles underlying the treatment is useful and in many cases almost specific for excitement and agitation. But to blindly put a patient into a pack because he or she is a nuisance on the ward and to leave the patient in for hours, struggling and noisy, is criminal, and if the case should ever come to court on the matter of malpractice it would undoubtedly get the physician who did such a thing into serious difficulty. Packs may be dangerous and every physician who has had prolonged experience in mental hospitals has noted instances of serious accidents which have occurred as a result of the pack. But in every case there has been one or more of the following deficiencies:

1. Lack of knowledge on the part of the physician of the physical condition of the patient and of his powers of reaction.
2. Deficiency of knowledge on the part of the physician of the technique and physiological action of the pack.
3. Carelessness on the part of the nurse in the pack room.
4. A nurse in charge who has not been properly trained.

In addition there are certain accidents that happen to patients in packs:

1. Heat exhaustion. Patients who are left in a pack for two or three hours at a time are always in danger of heat exhaustion. The symptoms of this are very clear and there is no excuse for such an accident.
2. Chilling. This occurs at times when the patient is left too long in the pack and proper precautions are not taken to prevent it.
3. Collapse. This is almost invariably due to some unsuspected heart condition and is usually due to lack of knowledge on the part of the physician as to the physical condition of his patient.

SECLUSION

Here again is a procedure which, when used intelligently in individual cases and for perfectly sound psychiatric reasons, may be a valuable way by which ward problems may be met. But the indiscriminate use of seclusion by ward nurses and attendants has resulted in many accidents in mental hospitals. To put the patient in a room by herself until the excitement has subsided is good therapy, but to leave a patient in a locked room hour after hour and day after day is abuse of the worst kind. When children become so irritable that they annoy others, seclusion in their own room may be a proper way of handling the situation. If psychotic patients have regressed to an infantile level of behavior, the same method may be indicated. Visits of the superintendent or a particular medical officer on the ward frequently cause certain patients to react violently. It is good therapy to place such a patient in a room by himself until the one who has disturbed him has left the ward. But this time should never extend beyond the time of the immediate emergency.

The use of all these procedures as a punishment for behavior that has occurred is decidedly unethical. It does no good, causes resentment in many patients, and is a misuse of a valuable method of psychiatric therapy.

Food

The food service of the psychiatric hospital is one of the most important morale-building factors in the institution, and can do more to retard or reinforce other therapeutic agencies than any other single administrative function. A normal man is difficult to feed without dissatisfaction, but the psychotic individual, with his distorted viewpoint on life, creates problems that are almost impossible to solve. Food is important to all human beings. A discussion of the different ways of solving the food problem cannot be given here, but any food service must take into consideration the preparation, variety, choice, service, temperature, and attractiveness of the food served.

There is a psychological side to the service. We do not eat only to live. A ritual has been built up around food service that is almost as important to most people as the food itself, and yet we do not always give the psychotic the credit of knowing what he is eating or even caring. Food service may be a therapeutic factor of great importance in the mental hospital.

There must be a rigid ward routine if the mental patient is not to slump down into deterioration. Such routine is calculated to keep the patient in the world of reality by having it impressed upon him and demanding his attention at all times. The success or failure of this program will always depend upon the enthusiasm and interest of psychiatrist, ward nurse, and attendant. Many traditional ways of carrying on custodial activities should be scrutinized carefully to eliminate and change the process in order to get the maximum amount of therapeutic efficiency. It is the abuse and not the use of seclusion and the wet pack that has thrown these useful adjuncts to therapy into disrepute. Destruction is a psychiatric matter. By careful studies of patients who destroy, ways and means can be devised to correct these destructive habits. Food is an important factor in custodial care. It can build morale, or tear it down. Administrators must take food service into serious consideration when setting up a therapeutic program. (Chart No. II).

CHART II.

THERAPY REPORT

Ward________________ Month________________ Nurse________________

Day of Month	1	2	3	4	5	6	7	8	9	10	11	12	13	14	15
GENERAL CARE															
Wash Face															
Brush Teeth															
Bath															
Trim Nails															
Toe-nails															
Shave															
Haircut															
Untidy-Bowels															
Urine															
Toileted-Bowels															
Enema															
Menstruation															
Beauty Parlor															
PHYSICAL ACTIVITIES															
Out-of-Doors															
Marching, Ward															
Calisthenics															
Dancing, Ward															
RECREATIONAL ACTIVITIES															
Ward Games															
Group Singing															
Group Reading															
Special Radio															
Library															
Books Given															
Church															
Dance															
Entertainment															
Party															
OCCUPATIONAL THERAPY															
Hospital Work															
Kitchen															
Sewing Room															
Industrial															
Laundry															
Dining Room															
Engineer															
Outside															
Others															
Ward Work															
Bed-Making															
Sweeping															
Dusting															
Toilets															
Bathroom															
Wash Windows															
Polishing															
Swabbing															
Linen															
Class Work, Ward															
Sewing															
Mending															
Arts & Crafts															
Other Work															
O. T. Center															

Chapter 6

THE MEDICAL AND SURGICAL SERVICE

The absorption of the psychiatrist in the problems of mental mechanisms, behavior manifestations, and situational relations is so complete in this day of dynamic psychiatry that he frequently fails to consider the fact that the patient has a physical body. The reports of mental hospitals which show causes of death might lead one to believe that mental patients do not have cancer, that tuberculosis is a rarity among them, and that nothing is physically wrong except cardiorenal conditions and senility. Yet mental patients are suspectible to physical disorders exactly as is the normal population. The careful psychiatrist who understands that the causation of a psychosis may be in any one or all of three fields—psychological, social, and physical—will not fail to take the soma into account in his study of the patient. The ship which leaves the dock with a skillful captain, good charts, and in a calm sea will not get very far if her hull is not seaworthy, her engines not running properly and her inter-communicating telegraph system not in good working order. The body is a part of the individual's environment and cannot be disregarded in any attempt to estimate the effect of that environment upon the mental life. The relationship existing between mind and body is too little understood for the psychiatrist to be careless in his consideration of physical disease.

Whether physical disorder has a specific effect in producing the psychoses has not, with a few exceptions, been proven, but these exceptions would indicate that the entire subject demands further research. But if physical disease does not, through specific channels, cause the psychoses, it cannot be denied that the reaction to illness may color and even change the symptomatic picture. Disease is not only a pathological process but an experience in life, and as with all experiences, the individual must adjust to it. This is relatively easy in minor illnesses but the reaction to serious conditions like cancer and tuberculosis is quite another matter.

For reasons such as those just discussed, a medical and surgical service is a necessity for a mental hospital. The purposes of such a service are:

A. *To give proper medical, surgical, and nursing care to all patients who develop, during the course of their psychosis, acute or chronic physical disease.*

Common humanity demands that we do everything possible for the patient who develops pneumonia, tuberculosis, cancer, or any other physical disorder. The minor accident rate in a mental hospital population is very high. Fractures are frequent and there is a considerable amount of surgery needed. The mental hospital administrator who values his public relationships will give much thought to the organization of proper medical and surgical facilities for his patients. Relatives who witness the careful work of well selected and thoroughly trained medical and nursing personnel during illness will be well pleased with the hospital, no matter what the outcome is. Such an organization is a splendid link with the community and indicates to relatives that the thing they can understand best—physical disease—is being properly attended to. An efficient medical department enhances the esteem in which the hospital is held by the medical profession.

B. *To study the effect of physical disease upon the psychoses and to trace the relationship that exists between the mind and body.*

Every practicing psychiatrist has noted instances of the complete cessation of mental symptoms during the course of an acute physical illness. What does this mean? The incidence of tuberculosis in the manic-depressive and schizophrenic psychoses needs elucidation. Does the psychosis contribute anything to the causation of the pathology or is the physical disease the cause of the psychosis? Is there any direct connection? What is the incidence of paranoid reaction types in patients suffering from pernicious anemia? What mechanisms are at work in bringing about the particular psychological reaction to that organic condition? What is the incidence of depressed, paranoid, and grandiose states in general paralysis? Is there any relationship between Kretschmer's body types and the psychotic manifestations of dementia paralytica? These and hundreds of similar questions can be answered only by the collaboration of the psychiatrist and internist.

C. *To make a complete physical inventory once each year of every patient in the hospital.*

How often do hospital psychiatrists find an inoperable cancer or a fully-developed case of tuberculosis which has progressed beyond the treatment stage? A careful and regular physical examination, with laboratory and X-ray studies, would have detected both conditions sufficiently early to have permitted remedial measures to be of some value. From a humanitarian point of view, if for no other reason, every mental hospital should be organized to protect its patients against the consequences of physical disease.

D. *To give a physical examination to every employee entering the service and check the health of the older ones at regular intervals.*

The health of the hospital employee after he has entered the service is a responsibility of the institution. It is economical to scrutinize his physical condition thoroughly before assuming this responsibility. The employee who has arteriosclerosis, a defective heart, or a kidney condition becomes an industrial risk when hired and may cause the State a great deal of expense for hospitalization and treatment. The employee who is not in good physical health is inefficient from the point of view of handling patients. He may be irritable, fault-finding, and even definitely paranoid as a result of physical disease.

E. *To care for employees of the hospital who develop acute illness.*

In spite of all precautions, the employee is subject to illness and the hospital is obligated to care for him. This care should be the best obtainable since the period of hospitalization, if prolonged, may be expensive. It is to the interest of the institution to get employees well as quickly as possible, and to do this it is essential that a proper organization be maintained.

ORGANIZATION

Specialization in medicine, while necessary, has had the practical effect of narrowing the interest of the specialist. He tends to treat an appendix, a heart, or a complex rather than a total organism. Every psychiatrist has seen cases in which eye specialists have tried to correct failing vision by refraction in a patient suffering from general paralysis. Surgeons have been guilty of operating upon hysterics, and psychiatrists have called the complaints of patients somatic delusions, until the patient finally died of cancer. There is no legitimate excuse for the specialist losing his interest in the individual. He may not have the necessary skill to go into other fields, but he should be sufficiently interested to utilize the assistance of technicians who are competent. The psychiatrist is rarely a good internist. Men who think in psychological terms tend to become so interested in tracing out the ramifications of a delusion or hallucination that they lose their skill as well as their interest in physical diagnosis. They may explain even physical symptoms on the basis of emotional conflict. Unfortunately this is frequently done without a careful physical study to exclude actual disease, and embarrassing situations have arisen in mental hospitals because of careless medical practice.

I am an advocate of a complete separation of the general hospital section of the mental hospital from the psychiatric service, at least in so far as routine work is concerned. This division would include the medical and nursing personnel. That this may not be taken too literally, I hasten to disclaim the idea that it should be so isolated that it is not available to the psychiatrist. It is really an adjunct to the psychiatric service and should be used by the psychiatrist exactly as he uses the pharmacy, hydrotherapy, or occupational therapy. It is a special division created for him to utilize in his study of the patient. Therefore it cannot be a distinct entity, except in an administrative sense. The chief of the service must have an understanding of the problems of the psychoses, even though his interests are primarily medical and surgical. He can never lose sight of the fact that his patients are in the hospital because of mental symptoms.

The psychiatrist must therefore use the service exactly as he would any professional department. Sending a patient to the medical and surgical wards for either study or actual treatment of disease does not relieve him of responsibility. The internist reports his findings to the psychiatrist and together they plan a therapeutic program. The evaluation of the relation of the physical findings to the psychiatric situation will always be the responsibility of the psychiatrist. He cannot evade it any more than he can shirk the responsibility for social service.

Unless the administrator is alert to the abuses that may creep into an organization of this type and unless he has a staff that is keenly interested in therapy, he may find the medical service degenerating into a "buck-passing" device. The psychiatrist sends the patient to a medical ward for study. The internist sends her back with the report, "physical findings negative," whereupon a difference of professional opinion comes into the picture and the patient suffers while physicians disagree. The very highest type of coöperation is essential in the efficient operation of a separate medical and surgical service. But in spite of such possibilities for disagreement, with a well-trained and enthusiastic staff, conferences between psychiatrist and internist will take the place of more independent attitudes. The internist works with the psychiatrist rather than for him, but the final decision is a psychiatric one. If the psychiatrists have had proper general training and the internists have had psychiatric experience, coöperation will be closer because of the respect of each for the problems of the other. It is equally essential that the medical nursing group have a thorough grounding in psychiatric as well as in general nursing technique.

LOCATION

The ideal location for a medical and surgical service is in a separate building which has been constructed for the purpose. It must be easily accessible from all parts of the hospital, and if the institution is widely scattered, an ambulance should be available. The service should not be housed in an admission building but should be in close proximity to it so that newly admitted patients may be adequately studied. It may not be possible to house the service in a separate building and the administrator will have to make the best use he can of his available space. If the institution is constructed on the cottage plan, one of the buildings may be adapted for the purpose. If the hospital is a Kirkbride institution, a group of wards must be set aside. The physical arrangement is largely a matter of finances. Special medical and nursing service can be carried on in any kind of building. The administrator who wishes to secure for his physically ill patients a better standard of medical and nursing care will not wait until a new building is constructed but will use the facilities he has at hand.

SIZE

A mental hospital with a capacity of 2,000 patients should reserve approximately 400 beds for physical disease. With this number, extra beds will always be available and no overcrowding will be present. They can be divided as follows:

Medical	100
Surgical	50
Neurological	50
Tubercular	50
Chronic disease	
Arteriosclerosis	
Senile conditions	140
Employees	10
Total	400

These figures are based on a study of the admissions to the medical and surgical service of the Worcester State Hospital over a period of ten years. Administrators who build for this purpose will find it necessary to establish a definite policy for such a service before deciding on bed capacity. If the wards are to be used only for incidental illness as it develops, a smaller capacity will meet the need. If it is to serve for the physical study of patients and for research in psychosomatic relationships, the capacity must be greater. But whatever policy is to be followed, all arteriosclerotic and decrepit senile patients should be housed on this service. For these patients separate wings are desirable, but since they are fundamentally medical and nursing problems they should be under the supervision of the medical service.

PERSONNEL

The ratio of physicians and nurses to patients must be a liberal one if the best type of care and treatment is to be given.

The ratio of physicians to patients should be 1-50. This would be divided as follows:—

Chief Internist
2 Senior Physicians
2 Junior Physicians
4 Graduate Internes

The chief internist should be a graduate of an approved medical school, have served a rotating internship of at least two years in an approved general hospital, and have had one year on the psychiatric service of a mental hospital. He must have marked administrative and organizing ability. Each assistant physician should have the same training as the chief of the service, with somewhat less experience.

The nursing personnel should be in charge of a chief supervisor who is responsible to the director of nursing. Each group of men's and women's wards are in direct charge of a supervisor throughout the twenty-four hours. General hospital graduates are preferable for these positions. But they should have had at least one year of postgraduate psychiatric training.

The ratio of ward personnel should be 1-5, divided as follows:

Medical	1—4
Surgical	1—3
Neurological	1—6
Tubercular	1—6
Chronic	1—8
Employees	1—4

These ratios do not take into consideration time off duty, illness, or vacations. They represent the number of nurses and attendants that should be on duty constantly.

The medical and surgical service of the mental hospital is a most important point of contact with the profession in the community. Here is where the general physician makes his contribution to the problem of mental disease and where he gets psychiatric experience. The visiting staff has not received the care and attention from administrators that it deserves. It has been the custom in many hospitals to appoint venerable physicians who are very jealous of their prerogatives but take their responsibilities lightly. If the members of this collaborating group are to make a real contribution they must be active and interested. How to secure this enthusiasm is a problem for the administrator. The prestige of the mental hospital has not yet reached the point where it is an asset to a physician to be on its staff. There is no material advantage for him unless he receives compensation. It is to be hoped that eventually the general profession will become so psychiatrically minded that service will be given as a contribution to public health. Hospitals located near metropolitan centers have less difficulty with this problem than those in rural communities. The former are able to secure visiting specialists who give freely of their time and energy. But in a rural community the visiting staff member must travel long distances and consume an inordinate amount of time to carry on his service. Here it becomes almost a necessity that he be reimbursed. Because of lack of funds, the amount of necessary medical work being done is reduced. This is particularly true of surgery.

A mental hospital of 2,000 beds and a yearly admission rate of 500, with an employee population of 600 and a well organized medical and surgical service, will have approximately 350 major surgical procedures each year if the necessary surgery is carried out. Most of this work will be done by visiting surgeons, but if it is not possible to have such an active subsidiary staff the administrator will have to organize his own surgical team. One cannot be sympathetic with those administrators who will not permit the resident staff to take any responsibility in medical and surgical matters. Such an attitude offers small encouragement to the young physician, fresh from a surgical internship, to come into the psychiatric hospital. Reckless surgery should not be permitted, but through careful selection of young physicians and offering the opportunity to gain medical and surgical experience, the mental hospital will be serving the patient more adequately.

The visiting staff should represent every branch of medicine. Two from each specialty may be appointed to serve for six-month periods. Records of their visits should be kept, and attendance at a monthly clinico-pathological conference should be part of their duties. If the hospital is to do its best work there must be a regular audit for both internist and psychiatrist. The visiting men must be an integral part of the staff and not simply physicians coming in as strangers to do a certain piece of work. The administrator must make every effort to build up staff loyalty among his visiting men. They must see themselves as part of the organization, if they are to give their best service.

ADJUNCT DIAGNOSTIC AND THERAPEUTIC FACILITIES

Surgical Unit

a. General Surgery
b. Orthopedic
c. Maternity

Special Clinics

a. Clinics
b. Radiology
c. Physical Therapy
d. Dental Unit
e. Eye, Ear, Nose, and Throat

GENERAL SURGERY

Operating Room. The heart of the surgical suite should be the operating room. It should embody modern construction and equipment. Good working tools are an incentive for every surgeon to take an interest in his responsibilities as a visiting staff member. If he gives his services he is entitled to the best equipment and well-trained personnel. The room should have an amphitheater for medical and nursing students, to accommodate approximately twenty.

Sterilizing Room. This should be of sufficient capacity to care for the sterilization requirements of the entire hospital. It should be located immediately adjacent to the operating room and the equipment must be of the most modern type. Antiquated instruments and sterilizers endanger the lives of patients, and no administrator can afford to take such a responsibility.

Anaesthesia Room. Modern surgery takes into account the psychological reactions of the patients. Careful preparatory technique is as necessary for psychiatric patients as it is for normal people. An attractively furnished anaesthesia room is indispensable in the surgical suite.

Surgeons' Room. Hospitals have not always considered the comfort and convenience of their visiting and resident surgeons. This room is an important factor in securing the services of active visiting men. It should contain lockers, shower, toilet and washing facilities, a small sitting room with comfortable chairs, smoking stands, and shelving for medical books.

Dictation Booth. This should be an alcove, sound-proofed and equipped with a dictaphone and telephone. The surgeon should dictate his notes immediately after coming from the operation or examination.

Scrub Room. This room should open off the operating room and be of sufficient size to take a double sink with a capacity for six people. This room may be used by both physicians and nurses.

Work and Linen Room. There must be sufficient shelving to take care of the linen in the surgical suite. This room should be at a distance from the operating room because of the necessity of keeping clean of lint and talcum.

Supply Room. A small room used for the storage of basins and utensils used in the operating room and adjacent to the latter.

Recovery Room. Should be a small ward with a capacity of four beds. It should have a blanket-warmer. Attractive decorations and furnishings in the room are an advantage.

Nurses' Office. This should have glass sides so the supervising nurse may have everything under her control. On one side the office should open into the instrument room and on the other side into a storage room for sterile material.

Instrument Room. All instruments must be under lock and key at all times. This room should have no entrance except through the office.

Gauze Storage Room. This room has only one entrance and that is through the office. All sterile material is stored in glass cases.

Nurses' Dressing Room. This need not be a large room but it should have lockers, toilets, and washing facilities.

Minor Surgery. This room should be well equipped for all minor surgery, accidents, and general treatments. Washing facilities are essential.

ORTHOPEDIC SURGERY

Plaster Room. The fractures occurring in a mental hospital are sufficiently numerous to justify special provision being made for their care. A Hawly table and sufficient space for plaster work would be all the equipment necessary for the room.

MATERNITY

This is not an essential part of the mental hospital medical and surgical service. In large state hospital systems it is desirable to send all delivery cases to one institution and that hospital should have adequate facilities for giving good care.

Delivery Room. This need not be a large room but should be equipped with a modern delivery table and other necessary accessories.

Wash Room. Opening off the delivery room should be a small room, with a sink for two people.

Nursery. A nursery for bassinets is indispensable for this suite. The capacity will depend upon the amount of work to be done.

CLINIC SUITES

An important part of a medical service is the maintenance of an out-patient and clinic service. The mental hospital is a community with a large population of patients and employees. Suitable facilities are an indispensable part of such a service.

Clinic Room. This should be for general clinic service. It is used for the diagnosis and treatment of gynecological, proctoscopic, and genito-urinary conditions. This would include diagnostic blood and spinal fluid tests and luetic treatments.

Eye, Ear, Nose, and Throat Room. This would require equipment used for the diagnosis and treatment of upper respiratory conditions and for testing vision.

Dental Office. This room should have at least two chairs, with sufficient space to increase the number to four when necessary.

Dental Laboratory. A small room for vulcanizing and other laboratory procedures should open from the dental office.

Room for Minor Surgery. This should have a capacity for approximately 50 cases for a population of 2,000. It is used for minor surgery, accidents, and general treatments.

Physician's Office. This should open directly from the general treatment room, and should be fitted with a desk, examining table, and filing cases for records.

Waiting Room. There should be two waiting rooms, one with a capacity for 40 patients and the other for 20. The larger is to be used for gynecological and dental clinics, the smaller one for the eye, ear, nose, and throat and the general clinic.

Dressing Room. These are cubicles which are used in conjunction with the large clinic room.

Toilet and Wash Room. This is for the use of patients. It should have at least two toilets and two lavatories.

Radiographic and Photographic Suite. This should be sufficiently large to take care of the best type of equipment.

Fluoroscopic Room. This should adjoin the general radiographic room.

Dark Room. This should have double equipment for both radiographic and general photographic work.

Interpreting Room and Office. This should be equipped with a viewing box and stereoscope.

Filing Storage Room. A fire-proof room adjoining the office and embodying the latest methods for safe film storage.

Waiting Room. A small room is sufficient.

PHYSIOTHERAPY

General Treatment. Should have an adequate amount of equipment, including facilities for the treatment of at least two general paretics at one time.

Muscle Re-Education. Equipped for mechanotherapy.

Hydrotherapy. This is used for special hydrotherapy as indicated in general medical and surgical conditions. It should be equipped with prolonged irrigation and whirlpool baths.

Office and Record Room. Should be located next to the general treatment room.

Waiting Room. A small room for patients who are to be treated.

All of these departments should be on one floor and close together. The personnel needed would of course depend upon the quantity of work to be done. The suite should be the responsibility of the director of nursing and in immediate charge of a well-trained surgical supervisor. She should have at least three graduate assistants, in addition to special technicians. There should be radiographic, physiotherapy, and dental technicians. A service of this kind cannot be efficiently managed from the general nursing office. If it is to function properly, technicians are necessary. No elaborate plant or physical equipment will take the place of well-trained personnel. In a suite of this capacity the amount of work carried on during the month should be adequate to care for the needs of a 2,000-bed mental hospital.

PHARMACY

General Drug and Dispensing Room. This should be sufficiently large to make proper dispensing possible.

Compounding Room. Opening off the drug room, there should be a compounding room where the pharmacist can properly prepare his prescriptions.

Manufacturing Room. This should be sufficiently large to permit the installation of suitable equipment for manufacturing on a reasonably large scale.

Narcotic and Alcohol Room or Vault. This should be connected with the general dispensing room, but it should be a room that can be securely locked up.

Supply Room. There should be two supply rooms. One of these is to be used for medicinal products and barrel storage. It would require a large-sized room. The other one should be in connection with it and should be for non-medicinal products, such as rubber goods.

Pharmacist's Office. Should have space for records.

LABORATORY DEPARTMENT

Routine Chemical Laboratory. A fairly large room, to be used as a work room for routine chemical work on patients.

Special Chemical Laboratory. This should be about the same size as the other but must be fully equipped with hoods and proper ventilating apparatus.

Basal Metabolism Rooms. There should be four rooms for basal metabolism determinations. These need be only large enough to contain a bed, chair, and the basal metabolism apparatus. It is important that such rooms be in a quiet location and be sound-proof.

PATHOLOGICAL LABORATORY

General Pathology. This is the ordinary general pathological workroom, and is a fairly large room.

Neuropathological Room. This should be about the same size as the other and sufficiently large to take the necessary equipment for work of this kind.

Microphotographic. Combined with a dark room.

Pathological Museum. This should be a sufficiently large room to house special specimens for permanent preservation.

Bacteriological Laboratory. This should be a fair-sized room and should contain the proper number of incubators to do the necessary work.

Sterilizing Room. This room is to be used for the purpose of sterilizing media and cleaning and preparing glassware for the pathologist.

Morgue. Equipped with automatic refrigeration and provision for eight bodies.

Autopsy Room. This should also have provisions for an amphitheater to seat twenty-five people.

Supply and Preserving Room. This is a room which is used for keeping supplies and specimens.

Physiological and Physical Laboratory. This should consist of three large rooms and is really for the purpose of providing for the future development of research in the laboratory section. They could be arranged so that they could be partitioned into small rooms.

Toilets. One for patients and one for employees.

Offices. There should be an office for the chemist, the chief technician, and the pathologist, and a large clerical office and record room.

Supply Rooms. Supply room for the entire laboratory suite. This should be a large space for supplies and chemicals and should be divided into three rooms, one for storage of chemicals, one for storage of glassware, and the third for storage of other supplies.

Dressing Rooms. Two dressing rooms for patients.

Waiting Room. There should be a waiting room for patients, to be used also as a receiving room for specimens.

ANIMALS

Animal House. This house or room should be sufficiently large to admit partitions being built to allow for the classification of animals. It is impossible to keep white mice and rabbits in the same room, and an adequate animal room should provide for this.

Janitor's Room. This is for the purpose of keeping food for animals, and supplies to be used in animal work. It should also have provision for cleaning material.

MEDICAL SERVICE ROUTINE

In any case where a patient shows physical symptoms and requires transfer to the medical service, the physician who wishes the transfer arranges for it with the chief of the service. He should give a history of the onset of the illness, the reason the patient is being sent, and a tentative diagnosis. This arrangement is usually carried out by telephone, but the referring physician incorporates all information in a signed statement which becomes a part of the medical record. The transfer is made by a supervisor upon orders from the head of the medical service.

Administrators may object to the "red tape" in this process, but I would point out that any procedure in the hospital should be carefully routinized in order that responsibility at any point may be definitely fixed. Orderly and systematic handling of these matters will not retard the service to the patient, unless personality clashes or incompetency are permitted to creep into the situation. The physician who is primarily interested in his own convenience rather than the welfare of the patient may utilize a system for his own selfish purpose, but this is always a problem of the administrator in every department of the hospital.

On the medical service the following procedure should be the first steps in the study of the illness:—

1. *Complete Blood Count.* The nurse in charge of the ward should order this by telephone, which order is later confirmed by the physician in writing. Good hospital practice demands that all orders from physicians be in writing. Nurses will be wise if they insist upon written orders in all cases because of the legal responsibility involved.

2. *Complete Urine Examination.* The nurse collects a urine sample and sends it directly to the laboratory without any special order.

3. *Temperature, Pulse, and Respiration.* The temperature, pulse, and respiration should be taken at once and properly charted.

MEDICAL RECORD

Good hospital practice calls for proper charting of medical data and no mental hospital can afford to be careless in this respect. The following record forms should be started by the nurse immediately upon the arrival of the patient on the ward. They are filed on the chart holder in the order given.

Clinical Chart. This is the standard temperature chart, and the pulse, temperature, and respiration should be recorded before the physician sees the patient.

Nurse's Notes. The nurse records the condition of the patient when he arrived on the ward. This note should include psychiatric observation, as well as physical condition.

Laboratory Sheet. As the reports come from the laboratory they are copied on the laboratory sheet for daily use.

Case History. A medical history should be taken by the physician and incorporated into the patient's records. A great deal of information may be obtained from the patient, but the psychiatric history always includes medical facts. The history and physical examination should be completed as quickly as possible.

Physical Examination. The physical examination should be carried out as quickly as possible after the patient arrives on the ward. A tentative diagnosis is recorded within twenty-four hours.

Continued Notes. The physician's observations should be made daily, at least during the acute stage of the illness.

Physician's Orders. Every order for treatment should be written and signed by the physician in charge of the patient.

Weight Chart. The weight of patients on the medical and surgical service should be taken at weekly intervals.

Statistical Card. This card is kept in a holder on the bed. It has the name, date admitted to the service, case number, ward from which patient was transferred, and physician who ordered the transfer. This is filled in by the nurse and serves as an identification of the patient. The remaining portion of the card consists of statistical information to be completed by the physician after the case is closed.

The statistical card is an important factor in the study of physical illness in its relation to mental disease. After the patient is discharged the card is sent to the record office, where a cross-index file may be maintained. Cards are filed under both mental and physical diagnoses. Without such a cross-index the information obtained from the medical service is of little value for study.

Consultations. Special consultations should be arranged for at any time and in any specialty. Where the service desired cannot be taken care of by the regular visiting staff, the administrative office should make the arrangement. A requisition is filled out by the physician requesting the service. This form is so arranged that the consultant may write his report on the back. It is then filed with the regular medical record.

Surgery. The senior physician in charge should make the final decision regarding major surgery. Before any operation can be performed, the nearest relative of the patient must give consent. This permission is required legally in most states. In cases of emergency where permission must be secured by telephone, it is always wise to have the operator listen to the conversation as a witness. The responsibility for surgical procedures rests entirely with the staff. Where surgical intervention is needed it should always be done. Where there are contraindications, no amount of scientific curiosity should be permitted to interfere with good surgical practice.

Administrators would do well to keep in mind the fact that the license to practice medicine carries the same responsibility in the hospital that it does in the community. Assistant physicians who are negligent in their work may find themselves in legal difficulties. There is no excuse for careless medical practice in the mental hospital. Low standards are due to neglect or lack of training on the part of individual staff members, and the fact should be emphasized that they and not the administrator carry the legal responsibility. In case this realization tends to make them timid and hence inactive in carrying on the necessary medical work, the hospital would be better off without them.

Danger List. When a patient's condition becomes so serious that death may be anticipated, his name is placed upon a "danger list" by the physician. When this occurs, two very important responsibilities immediately fall on the physician. The nearest relative should be notified and the religious needs of the patient taken care of. The former should be notified by telephone or telegraph and the chaplain by telephone. Much unpleasant criticism has resulted from carelessness of hospitals in these respects. Every physician should understand the importance of carrying out the rules in regard to such procedures. The administrator has to bear the criticism that comes from continued negligence in these important matters, and eventually the hospital will suffer in prestige.

Deaths. When death occurs the physician is notified immediately, and he should proceed at once to the ward and pronounce the patient dead. Too much care cannot be exercised in safeguarding patients on the ward from the knowledge of what is happening. Patients whose death is expected should be moved to a room or a cubicle. Every reverence should be shown. The callousness with which death is treated in some hospitals is repugnant to patients and disgusting to most normal people. Negligence or carelessness in this respect on the part of either nurse or physician should not be tolerated. Civilization decrees that our dead shall be treated with respect. This attitude should be conspicuously reflected in the institution where other patients may receive considerable hurt from the effect of sights which indicate a disregard for conventions. A mortuary report, noting bruises or discoloration of the body, should be made out by the physician. There should be a space for the signature of everyone who handles the body—the physician, the supervisor, and the undertaker who receives it. This fixes responsibility. Too much care cannot be exercised with regard to identification. Many embarrassing mistakes have been made in hospitals, and every precaution should be taken to mark the remains properly and to avoid any exchange of tags or identification marks.

It is essential that relatives be notified immediately when death has occurred. Here is another point at which carelessness frequently creeps in. It should be an invariable rule of every hospital that relatives be called immediately by telephone after death has occurred. If this is not possible, the telegraph should be used. It is at this time that permission for autopsy is requested.

Relatives visiting patients whose names are on the danger list should receive every courtesy and consideration. Of course this is true of all visitors to the hospital, but when death is imminent the obligation of the hospital is particularly important. Serving refreshments to them, permitting them to remain overnight in a comfortable room, and assisting them in every way possible, is not only a humane attitude to take but will make friends for the hospital.

Autopsies. The scientific efficiency of the modern hospital is judged to a considerable degree by the autopsy rate. This is as it should be. It is largely by the study of the pathology of disease that new facts will be obtained for the use of the clinician. But a large percentage of autopsies means more than interest and enthusiasm on the part of the clinical staff. The autopsy percentage is in direct proportion to the confidence and good will the hospital has built up among the relatives of patients. If these people believe that the medical and nursing staff has had a real interest in the patient and if all members of the organization with whom they have come in contact have shown a spirit of sympathy and kindliness, the request for an autopsy will invariably result in the required permission. The autopsy rate of any hospital is therefore one index of the standing it has in the community. The permission is the culmination of a long series of pleasant relationships between the hospital and that section of the community represented by the family of the patient. Autopsy permission should always be obtained in writing when possible. When telephone permission is obtained, the operator should be instructed to listen to the conversation in order that a witness may be available, if needed. In case no relatives are found, interment will usually take place in the hospital cemetery. Administrators would do well to give some thought to the procedure in these state funerals. Here again any disregard of modern customs may react disastrously on the institution. Religious services should be carried out with a properly qualified clergyman in attendance and with all the ritual and reverence that modern society decrees in such a situation.

Medico-Legal Cases. The mental hospital administrator should protect his hospital from any possible criticism by calling into consultation the proper legal officer in any case of violent death. One should be over-scrupulous in these matters. The following are some of the cases which call for such procedure:

All cases of patients who die within forty-eight hours after admission to the hospital;

Those having had a fracture within a period of twelve months preceding the death;

Case of unexpected death;

Case of suicide, accidental death, or a death of obscure origin;

Any death following an accident or fight in which employees have been involved;

Any case where there are suspicious circumstances.

Employees' Clinic. The responsibility for the care and treatment of hospital employees is a grave one for the administrator. A complete record of the examination and treatment of every employee who is ill should be an inflexible rule. This is particularly essential in states which have industrial accident indemnity laws. The efficient way of handling this matter is by a daily employees' clinic, held at a regular hour. At this clinic any employee who needs attention for physical sickness should be treated and a careful record made. A monthly summary should be prepared for the administrator. A study of these will indicate employees who are costing the hospital an excessive amount for medical treatment. It should be a rigid rule that no casual prescribing will be permitted except where an actual emergency exists.

Employees' Physical Examination. New employees should be given a careful physical examination. It is preferable to do this before the individual is assigned to duty, but if this is not possible, the employment should be contingent upon the results of the examination. This physical survey should emphasize the condition of the respiratory tract, tests of sight and hearing, superficial neurological tests, and the external abdominal rings. In addition to the examination, every employee should be given typhoid, paratyphoid, and smallpox vaccine, unless he can produce written evidence that successful inoculation has been completed within three years. Some hospitals perform a Wassermann test on all new employees.

Surgical Operations. The question as to whether the hospital is obligated to care for its employees surgically is rather an involved one. It would seem that there can be no general rule about the matter. Each case will have to be judged on its own merits. Common sense must be used in deciding, always keeping in mind that anything that will contribute to the well-being of good employees is worth the cost.

Administrative Checks. The work of the medical and surgical service lends itself to an administrative checking system better than many other departments of the hospital. A system of records which can be summarized into a monthly report for the administrator will give him a picture of the activity of the service. If these reports are transferred to graphs he will have a topic for discussion with the staff that will do much to keep the entire group up to a high standard of accomplishment.

Movement of Population. The record of patients admitted to and discharged from the service is important.

Discharges Detailed as to Physical Condition. This shows patients who were discharged recovered, improved, not improved, not treated, and dead.

DEATHS DETAILED

Number of Medico-legal cases
Number of Autopsies
Autopsies confirmed ante mortem diagnoses
Autopsies partially confirmed ante mortem diagnoses
Autopsies refuted ante mortem diagnoses
Attendance at autopsies
Primary causes of death
Average age of death

CONSULTATIONS DETAILED

Eye
Ear, Nose, and Throat
Gynecological
Medical
Orthopedic
Radiography
Others

Only members of the visiting or courtesy staff are noted on this report.

DETAILED SURGERY

Major Operations
Minor Operations
Total

CLINIC EXAMINATIONS	*Number*	*Patients*
Eye Examinations	"	"
Ear, Nose, and Throat	"	"
Gynecological	"	"
Luetic Treatment	"	"
Smallpox Vaccinations	"	"
Spinal Punctures	"	"
Typhoid and Paratyphoid inoculations	"	"
Wassermanns	"	"
Others	"	"

DRESSINGS (*Outpatient*)

Abrasions and Lacerations
Boils and Carbuncles
Burns
Infections
Ulcerations
Others
Total Outpatient Dressings
Ward Dressings

OCCUPATIONAL THERAPY

Patients receiving O.T. on Wards
Patients receiving O.T. Outside

EMPLOYEES' CLINIC

Number of Physical Examinations of new employees
Number of food handlers examined and cultured
Examined and treated at clinic
Required hospitalization
Required operation
Total days on sick ward

LABORATORY REPORT

Give number of times each procedure was performed

PATHOLOGICAL REPORT

Tissue specimens (Surgical)
Tissue Sections (postmortem)
Classification of tissue

RADIOGRAPHIC DEPARTMENT

Part Examined
Give number of plates and patients

PHOTOGRAPHY

Photographs
Lantern Slides
Photomicrographs
Motion Picture Films

DENTAL DEPARTMENT

Apiectomy
Bridges
Cleanings
Examinations (routine)
Extractions
Fillings
Microscopic Examinations
Plates
Repairs
Treatments
X-ray Diagnoses
Others
Total examinations and treatments
Total patients examined and treated
Total general anaesthetic cases

PHYSICAL THERAPY

Classification of Treatments and Tests
Total Treatments and Tests
New Patients Received During Month
Total Patients Treated
Classification of Diseases.

The medical and surgical service should be considered as an adjunct to the psychiatric care of the patients and not as a distinct entity entirely divorced from psychiatry. Its head should therefore be sympathetic towards and have an understanding of the problems and objects of psychiatry. The material on this service should be utilized to some extent for clinical investigation. All medical and surgical work should be coordinated under this service. The treatment of luetic patients, the treatments by means of physiotherapeutic equipment, X-ray therapy, etc., should thus be under the supervision of the Medical-Surgical Service. Much of the teaching activities of nurses and medical students are given on the wards of this service, and opportunity for introduction to psychiatric aims should be utilized. The student should be shown that a patient is not simply a disoriented organic mechanism but a human being. The head of this service should utilize to the fullest extent the special technical skill and training of all the various members of the staff.

Many may object to such a type of organization on the basis that it shuts out the psychiatrist from medical work. This is true if the psychiatrist is sufficiently disinterested to be shut out. But if he is a physician who sees the need of the expert assistant in his study of a patient, he will welcome such an arrangement and will utilize it to the fullest extent.

Chapter 7

GROUP PSYCHOTHERAPY

THE purpose behind the attempt to build morale among normal people is to move the group towards a single purpose rather than a diversity of goals. Management endeavors to mold and change the ideals of individuals so that they may act as an integrated organism rather than as single units. The goal towards which the group is moving must be implanted by management. Group purpose rarely generates spontaneously. It becomes operative in proportion to the organized efforts made by leaders to create it. The methods and techniques by which a unity of purpose may be brought about are of interest to every employer of labor.

The mental hospital administrator has this problem with patients. Building morale becomes a system of therapy through the power of suggestion. To one who raises the argument that psychotic patients cannot be reached by the means that the employer of labor uses, I should answer, "Have we ever tried to apply the multiplicity of techniques that modern business has used so effectively, as a therapeutic weapon in the rehabilitation of a group of psychotics?"

Obviously the state will never be able to furnish a sufficient number of psychotherapists to treat patients on an individual basis. Even if the cost were not prohibitive, the trained personnel could not be obtained at the present time. The administration must step in and reinforce the efforts of individual psychiatrists by organized re-educational efforts. This is what is meant by group psychotherapy, in its broadest sense.

The problem with psychotics is in some respects of greater complexity than that which confronts the employer of labor. The patient is asocial and the powerful factor of contagion does not act as readily as in a normal group. Despite this, however, ward social standards are effective in molding the behavior of individual patients.

The constant exposure of patients on all sides and in all

ways to suggestion will bring them into closer harmony with the hospital and lead to better behavior. Administration organized around the idea of trying to improve morale through direct and indirect suggestion will change the atmosphere of the hospital. The effort to make reality so insistent that the patient cannot get away from it is a type of group psychotherapy that should be used more widely than it is. If the superintendent can create an attitude of coöperation and a belief that the hospital is a place of good will and fair play, group spirit will be a powerful factor in the recovery of the individual.

In the attempt to change the patient-hospital relationship it is effective to make use of the devices that the commercial world finds of value in creating a desire for a particular product. Educational propaganda has transformed the thinking of nations. It has swayed the emotions of thousands and through it great fortunes have come into existence. Allowing for the difference in the susceptibility to suggestion between the psychotic patient and the normal individual, it seems reasonable to believe that a modification of the same methods may be used to build morale among mental hospital patients.

In planning group psychotherapy through educational propaganda it is important that the administrator know exactly what he wishes to accomplish. We cannot sell the product, mental health, unless we know exactly what we are offering.

1. *Acceptance of Reality.* If reality constantly presses in upon a patient, sooner or later he accepts it, at least in part. But it must be sufficiently unusual and changing so that his acceptance will not become automatic.

2. *Confidence in the Hospital.* If the best hospital-patient relationship is to exist, the patient must have a belief in the good intentions of the institution. He must not only be constantly told that everything is for his benefit, but the acts of every person who comes in contact with him must show that this is true.

3. *Tolerance for Others.* The psychotic fails at the social level of life. His withdrawal from reality includes an abstinence from social relationships. Restoration of his ability to fraternize with others must be a main goal in any attempt to rehabilitate him.

4. *Personal Appearance.* The absorption in his dream world makes the psychotic neglect his personal appearance. This is intensified by a lack of good standards in the patient group with which he is associated. If there is no social pressure to be neat and clean, few patients will maintain good standards of their own initiative.

5. *Interest in an Occupation.* It is a matter of common knowledge that men accept the discipline and responsibility of occupation more readily than women. They have generations of orderly, disciplined work behind them, while women have always been employed in the home without supervision. Therefore they respond less readily.

6. *Ability to Play.* The pleasurable emotion generated by play is not strong in the psychotic. Yet the play instinct is a powerful factor in the life of human beings.

These are the goals to be attained through the creation of a hospital group spirit. The program of mass therapy must be built around attempts to strengthen the power of each patient to see the importance of each object and make a real effort to achieve it. All propaganda makes use of suggestion. Industrialists have been very ingenious in devising ways and means by which direct and indirect suggestion is projected into the homes of American people.

McDougall [24] says that suggestion is a process of communication resulting in the acceptance, with conviction, of the communicated proposition, independently of the subject's appreciation of any logical grounds for its acceptance.

The acceptance of a suggestion depends, to a considerable extent, upon the belief on the part of the subject in the superior knowledge, broad understanding, or actual authority of the one making the suggestion.

The patient may accept a suggestion from the ward psychiatrist because the latter is a physician and the patient shares the belief of modern society that physicians are men of superior knowledge. He may accept it from the nurse because he thinks she understands his problems better than anyone else. And finally he may accept it from the superintendent as one in authority. If all these individuals suggest the same thing the patient will eventually respond.

Conscious suggestion is increased by attention on the part of the subject. Psychotics have a high threshold of consciousness. It is difficult to get their attention except through special means. The degree of attention that the psychotic is giving at any time is difficult to estimate. Apparently when they are furthest from reality more facts are registered than one would think.

The more social the group the greater is the suggestibility. The extroverted manic responds more quickly to group action than does the introverted schizophrenic. Building up group attitudes will aid in suggestion to the individual patient. If we can reinforce the suggestion of brushing the teeth by having the patient see everyone else do it, and if other patients will tell him it is the thing to do, we get the effect of group suggestion.

Normals act on suggestion constantly. Every store window, every person we pass on the street, everyone we meet conveys positive or negative suggestion to us. We are constantly confronted by the suggestion that this or that thing will bring us material profit or emotional satisfaction. The more people we meet the more suggestion we get.

Women are more suggestible than men. A strong concentration of effort to utilize therapeutic suggestion on the women's wards is badly needed in the mental hospital. But women are more individualistic than men and one gets less assistance from the group.

The young are more suggestible than the old. The fixity of ideas in the latter prevents much flexibility.

The better informed the patient is about the matter that is to be impressed on his mind the less suggestible he is. If he has been told by the physician that the hospital will not permit him to be unkindly treated by any attendant and the patient knows by experience that attendants do treat patients improperly, he will not accept the suggestion. He knows more about the matter than the physician.

Suggestibility varies in the individual as it changes in the group. Even psychotics follow the crowd within narrow limits. Occupation may be approved or disapproved by the majority of patients on a ward. If the latter is the case it is difficult to get any patient interested in occupation.

How to utilize these psychological principles in therapy is a problem of the administrator. It should be his chief concern. Suggestion may be conveyed through the spoken and written word, through sight, sound, taste, and smell. Man has devised countless ways to disseminate it. I can only mention briefly a few of the ways in which it can be turned to account in the treatment of psychiatric patients.

THE WRITTEN WORD

How can we make suggestions through writing? Is this a practical way of building patient morale? Will the patient react emotionally to a written communication?

The time for beginning a program of group suggestion is the moment the patient enters the hospital. Organized propaganda, educational in its purpose, should greet him when he is received and continue throughout his residence. The admission letter has proved to be of value in strengthening the initial rapport. The letter is delivered to the patient as soon as he is comfortably settled in bed. The nurse remains until he reads the letter and explains any point on which he is not clear. The original letter used at this hospital was a general one, but following a careful study of patient reaction by Dembo and Hanfmann [25] a revision was made and it is now used in the following form:

Dear ————

I am sending you this letter in the hope that it may help you to get your bearings in this new and unusual situation. I know how confused anyone must be in coming to this hospital for the first time. The place is so large, there are so many people about, and there are so many different ways of doing things that it is hard to get matters straight.

Because of this, I am sending you, together with this letter, some information about the way of doing things here that I hope will help you. It is hard to think in advance of all the questions you may want to ask, but I am sure that everyone in the hospital will be glad to give you any information that is not given in this leaflet. Do not hesitate to ask questions about things you do not understand.

As the Superintendent of the hospital I extend to you my greetings. I want you to know that we are interested in your comfort and well-being while you are here. But more than this—we are most anxious to help you in every way to make your time in the hospital as short as possible. I hope you will profit by your stay here and that you will leave with feelings of friendship towards the institution.

There are 2200 patients in this hospital. I cannot, therefore, know each one as intimately as I should like, but there are many doctors, nurses, and other assistants, who are as anxious to help you as I am. I hope you will have full confidence in them. You may also write a personal letter to me if you think there is any special thing I can do for your comfort and well-being.

Cordially yours,

Superintendent

INFORMATION ABOUT HOSPITAL

The questions in this leaflet have been asked by patients admitted to this hospital over a period of many years. If you will read the pamphlet carefully the information in it will help you understand why you are here. The nurse will tell you in greater detail about those matters upon which you wish further explanation.

1. *What is this place?* It is a hospital maintained by the State for the cure of people who have mental or nervous illness. It is located in the city of Worcester and is the largest of eleven State hospitals. There are 2200 patients here, and 500 employees.

2. *Why are people brought here?* People are usually brought here because someone in the community thought that their ideas and actions were very strange and reasoned from this that their mind must be sick. It may have been friends, relatives, or even a stranger. People are sent here to find out whether or not they are ill.

3. *How long do people stay here?* That depends entirely upon what the doctors find. If they do not believe that you have any sickness that should cause you trouble, you may leave just as soon as they decide. But if they find you are ill, then you must remain until you are better. Your doctor will be glad to talk it over with you.

4. *Can one write letters?* Certainly. Ask the nurse for paper, envelopes, and pencil. Please leave your letters unsealed. The law says that the doctor must read all mail leaving the hospital, but we always send the letters if they are not indecent or threatening. Of course, all letters sent to you will be given to you unopened.

5. *How can patients take care of their affairs outside the hospital?* There are specially trained social workers in the hospital who will see the people outside of the hospital about business that patients may have. They may also be helpful to patients in making all necessary arrangements for the time when they leave the hospital.

6. *When can relatives and friends come to see patients?* The regular visiting days are Tuesday, Saturday, and Sunday of each week. All holidays are also visiting days. The hours are from 9 to 11 in the morning, and from 1:30 to 4:30 in the afternoon.

7. *Why are new patients kept in bathrobes?* For two reasons. First—to enable the doctor to carry out a careful physical examination and to do certain tests. Second—to give the office a chance to list and mark your clothes so they will not be lost. They are usually returned after two or three days.

8. *What happens to the patient's money?* Any money that the patients bring to the hospital or any that is sent by their relatives is deposited in the Treasurer's office, where it is kept safe for the use of the patient.

9. *Can one buy things in the hospital?* Yes, there is a store in the hospital, and patients can buy what they want with their money, if the doctor approves the order. The nurse will prepare a list of store orders every once in a while, usually on Saturday or Sunday. Tell her what you want, and she will put in an order for the Treasurer to pay for it out of your money.

10. *Can one smoke?* Certainly, if one wants to and if one's health permits. Ask the nurse to take you to a place where smoking is permitted and give you a light.

11. *Are there any entertainments in the hospital?* During the fall and the winter time there are picture shows on Wednesdays and dances every once in a while. Ask the nurse to take you to them. In the summer there are games and concerts.

12. *Can one go out for walks?* There are seven wards on the men's side and six on the women's side that have no locked doors. Patients on these open wards have ground privileges, which means

that they are free to come and go on the grounds as are the employees. They are permitted to go to the city at certain times, and frequently go home to spend a few days. Ground privileges are given to patients only if they behave in a normal and sensible way, and consent to follow certain rules. Your doctor can tell you about these rules. To be placed on an open ward is a step towards home.

13. *How does one get books to read?* Ask the nurse to take you to the library or get a book for you. We have an excellent library which we hope you will use.

14. *Does one have a chance to go to church?* Yes. We have Catholic services each Sunday morning at 9, Protestant services at 10:15, Jewish service twice each month on Sunday afternoon, and Episcopal service once each month. We have both a Catholic and Protestant chaplain attached to the hospital.

15. *What is going to happen during the next few days?* Your doctor will have long talks with you and ask you many questions about yourself and your family. You will also be given a thorough physical examination. Your eyes, nose, and throat will be examined; some blood will be taken from your arm for analysis, and your teeth will be examined in the dental office. After all the examinations have been completed, the doctors will discuss in a staff meeting whether something should be done for you in the hospital, or whether you are well enough to go home.

16. *How can one spend one's time in the hospital?* Ask the nurse if she can find any occupation for you on the ward. If you want any other occupation, ask for the O.T. girl. We say O.T. for Occupational Therapist. They are specially trained people who can teach you new and interesting occupations. You can tell them by their dress: they wear bright blue uniforms, and no caps.

17. *What good does one get from occupation?* Occupation keeps the troublesome thoughts away, keeps you interested in useful things, and gives the necessary exercise to your mind and body. Work for your own sake and peace of mind if your doctor finds that you are physically able. To take an interest in some occupation is the best and quickest way to convince the doctors that you are well enough to go home.

18. *Do many patients leave this hospital?* Each year about 500 patients are discharged from the hospital. We need room for so many new patients coming in all the time, that we are only

too glad to send a patient home as soon as we can. Listen to the radio on the ward, and once each month you will hear the names of the patients who have been discharged from the hospital during the month.

It was found from the study that 69 out of 100 patients read and understood the letter, either wholly or in part. The effect in the great majority of cases was a positive one. It was appreciated mainly as a source of information about the basic facts of hospitalization and life in the hospital. By enabling the patient to orient himself in his new situation, it helped in relieving his uncertainty and apprehension. Other but not less valuable functions were those of giving him practical directions for his behavior and of restoring his self-respect. The latter was produced less by the contents of the letter than by the fact that the general tone was one of consideration for him.

Other letters can be sent to the newly admitted patient at intervals of several days to a week, each one reinforcing the original but presenting the material in a different way. The second communication might contain more detailed information regarding legal methods of commitment. Patients are always interested in this subject, and I know of nothing on which they show greater confusion. A third letter giving details about the different departments of the hospital would be helpful. The number of tons of coal used, the number of loaves of bread baked, etc., would show that the patient was in a large institution. In this country we are impressed by bigness. One of the points noted in the study was that most patients were overwhelmed, impressed, and even pleased by the size of the hospital to which they had come, though involuntarily.

Most patients are more or less apprehensive about the staff conference where their case is to be considered. They think of the proceeding as a court. A letter can be delivered before the patient has this experience, giving information about the meeting and telling what will occur. There are many variations of this plan. Naturally the information given will change with the individual hospital. The questions and answers can be put into an attractively illustrated booklet. A freshly written communication actually signed by the superintendent would be excellent if the admission rate were not too large. The more personal these are, the more powerful they become in building morale.

Other communications can be sent to the patient from the office of the superintendent. Frequently letters come from relatives stating that the patient does not write. A note of reminder to the patient may stimulate him to do so and it will certainly give him considerable satisfaction to receive it.

It would be excellent therapy for the administrative office to notify the patient every time an inquiry is received from his home. Such a letter can be a regular form but always freshly written.

The following are indicative of the kind of communications that bring rich returns in the form of better hospital-patient rapport:

My dear Mr. Doe,

We have today received a letter from your (Relative) asking about your mental and physical health. Why not write and tell her about yourself? I know she will appreciate hearing from you.

Sincerely,

Superintendent.

A letter should be sent to the patient when money is received, informing him of the fact.

My dear Mr. Doe,

We have today received (Amount) from your (Relative), which is to be used for (Purpose). The money has been placed to your credit in the Treasurer's Office.

Please write your (Relative) and thank her for this money.

Sincerely,

Superintendent.

It is an excellent practice for the superintendent to answer the communications of patients. Most of them find their way into the waste basket. Psychotic patients get many delusions about their letters, and great care is needed to prevent these ideas from having a real foundation in fact. Every ward in the mental hospital should have a locked mail box where a patient may drop his letters. These boxes should be made as nearly like the official United States mail receptacles as possible. Putting a letter into such a box gives the patient a sense of security about his mail that he cannot have when he has to coax a supervisor to take it. There is much carelessness in many mental hospitals about taking care of out-going letters written by patients. If a letter is not sent it should be returned to the writer with a written explanation giving the reasons why it has not been mailed. Absolute honesty with patients is an excellent builder of morale.

When the superintendent answers the patient by correspondence his answer should be noncommittal. Any attempt to particularize may lead to difficulty.

Such a form letter would be:

Dear Mrs. Doe,

I have received your note of (Date). Thanks for writing me. I shall be glad to go over the matter with you the next time I visit your ward.

Sincerely,

Superintendent.

And he must be sure to see her when he does visit the ward, or the letter will do more harm than good.

Booklets. Many booklets and pamphlets containing mental hygiene material can be distributed to patients. These must be written down to the level of the average individual and some of them should be in languages other than English. A copy of each booklet can be sent to the patient at regular intervals.

The Hospital Paper. Hospitals frequently distribute a weekly or monthly paper to the wards. My objection to many of them is that they deal entirely with hospital gossip. Such a paper should be carefully planned to attract the patient's attention and at the same time present some mental hygiene material. Articles on nursing, occupational therapy, hydrotherapy, and general medicine should be published. Official hospital statistics are interesting—number of patients leaving the hospital, jobs in hospital industry where patients can work, and stories dealing with institution life. It should be written in newspaper style and not in heavy medical or psychiatric phraseology. A weekly issue is preferable and a sufficient number should be printed for distribution to everyone. It would be particularly valuable if they could be addressed directly to the patient on an addressograph machine. The editorship of such a paper cannot be carried on by patients. It must be done by someone who can be held to a measure of responsibility by the administrator.

Hospital Pictorial. This is an illustrated weekly which consists entirely of pictures of the hospital. New personnel, new equipment, new construction, pictures of the gardens, and similar subjects can be used. Several of these are hung on each ward bulletin board.

LIBRARY

Most mental hospitals have a library for the use of patients. But an indiscriminate collection of books housed in a room does not constitute a library. Nor does such a library do much good in treatment. There are three factors necessary to make a therapeutic library:

The Books. Books have no value as a therapeutic agent unless they are carefully selected. I have known hospital libraries where the administrator bought books in lots of 100 simply because they were cheap. Books do affect our lives, and while it may be true that the majority of our patients are not extensive readers, they should be urged to read the kind of books that are suited to their psychological needs—books that teach lessons in healthy thought and normal action, books that exemplify the homely virtues, books that bring out lessons of courage to face reality. Bibliotherapy is more than a mere name. It is really a factor of great importance when properly used. But books should be selected and prescribed with as much care by the psychiatrist as he would use in selecting and prescribing the drugs he uses. In psychiatry they are of more importance than the drugs.

The Librarian. The second essential is a good librarian—not an individual whose conception of her function is to see that the books are kept in repair and are not stolen but one who believes that her business is to induce patients to read the kind of books the psychiatrist wants them to read, the kind of books that will help them solve their problems. She should see herself as the technical assistant of the psychiatrist. Such a librarian will be an asset to the hospital. She will be well educated in library technique but she will also be trained in normal and abnormal psychology and in actual work with psychotics. Psychiatric bibliotherapy will be a specialty and a career for her. She will have a personality that will permit her to work in harmony with and as an aide in the psychiatric team. She will see the library in its proper relation to other methods of treatment, neither over- nor under-estimating its importance in the therapeutic scheme. She will realize that the library is the intellectual pharmacy of the hospital.

The Place. A central library where patients may come and read is also an essential part of this program. Such a room furnishes a place where they can meet and get on terms of better social relationship. It should be easily accessible and attractively furnished. Libraries are rarely planned in any building scheme. They are usually tucked away in some corner that can best be spared and without regard for their accessibility and convenience.

In addition to this central library, a branch should be maintained on each side of the hospital. Where the institution is built on the cottage plan there should be one to each group of cottages. These should be accessible to the closed wards. The more difficult books are to obtain, the less they will be used by patients. Each branch is presided over by a student librarian or a nurse who has some interest and understanding. The general supervision is given by the librarian. Branch libraries need not be large but each should have at least 100 books and a book cart. They should be opened only when the librarian is not on the wards with the truck. Books must be brought to patients; they will not come to the books unless urged.

Pictures. The mental hospital has a considerable amount of blank wall space on each ward that can be put to good use in suggestive education. I do not advocate imitating our American roads, but attractive signs would be decorative and informative. The following signs, attractively made up, help to create good will among patients:

Time of Church Service
Visiting Days
Library Hours
Rules of Mental Health
Forms of Commitment
Ward Routine
Obligations of a Parole Ward
Rules for Smoking
Explanation of Hydrotherapy
Occupational Therapy

If an attractive set of posters could be made up which would be of some psychological significance to the patient, they would do more good than the old-fashioned woodcuts and steel engravings that decorate the wards of our older mental hospitals. These may be valuable to collectors or art enthusiasts but are of no help in treating the psychoses. I thoroughly believe in attractive pictures, but they may as well be designed to help the patient as to be just pictures. Why not suggest something to him with ward decorations? Pictures of scenes in and about the institution are valuable. They can be identified by the patient, and he familiarizes himself with his environment.

Bulletin Boards. Every ward in the mental hospital should have a bulletin board. On this are posted the following:

Hospital Pictorial
Schedule of Entertainments
Radio Programs
Winners of Contest Tournaments
New Inter-ward Contests
Patients Going Home
Mental Hygiene Suggestions
New Books
Clippings from Newspapers
Hospital News

Stereopticon Slides. These may be used at the moving picture show to drive home suggestions, attract attention, and arouse interest. They can also be used for community songs. The following have been used to create interest in contests:

> A STORY CONTEST
> DO YOU KNOW ANY GOOD STORIES?
>
> If you do, send them to the radio room. For every story shown on the screen a prize will be awarded.

> SEND IN A STORY TODAY
> DO YOU WANT TO WIN A PRIZE?
>
> If you do, watch these slides and find out exactly how it can be done.

> HOW WELL DO YOU KNOW THIS HOSPITAL?
>
> Can you recognize the people here? Do you know who your neighbor is? Can you tell what the buildings are used for? Are you interested in these things?
>
> WATCH CLOSELY—THINK HARD

> THIS IS THE WAY TO WIN A PRIZE
>
> At every entertainment we shall show a picture of someone in the hospital, a department of it, or a scene that you should recognize. To the patient who names the three correctly, we shall give a prize.
>
> YOU CAN WIN A PRIZE!

WATCH CLOSELY—THINK HARD
WHO IS THIS?

A picture of the Superintendent.

WHAT BUILDING IS THIS?

A picture of front of hospital.

WHAT PLACE IS THIS?

Picture of Cafeteria.

A REMINDER

Have you written a letter home this week?

IF NOT DO IT TOMORROW

Tell them how you are. The folks at home want to hear from you.

GOING HOME

Do patients ever go home from the hospital?

This question is asked many times.

HERE IS THE ANSWER

Discharged from hospital 450 in 1935.

THEY RECOVERED

So can you.

INCOMING LETTERS TO PATIENTS

Even this can be used for the purpose of suggestion. It would take only a short time to attach a sticker to each letter when the mail is being distributed, on which is a printed suggestion.

BE SURE TO ANSWER THIS LETTER The folks at home want to hear from you. Write now.

DON'T FORGET The entertainment tonight. You will enjoy it.

LISTEN TO THE RADIO Each evening at 6:45 there is a message to you.

These stickers should be changed at least once a week. A dozen sets can be printed and if one set is used each week the series can be repeated several times. Many kinds of information can be disseminated in this way. Advertising? Of course it is advertising, but it is also group therapy. It is positive suggestion. It brings some patients back to reality. Undignified, perhaps, but less dignity and more effort to cure patients with whatever means are at hand would bring results.

THE SPOKEN WORD

The lecture is still a good way to disseminate information. We psychiatrists spend much time telling the community how to live. How much time do we spend telling our patients about themselves? A series of talks on mental disease and health would attract more patients than one would think. Let us not assume that our patients are incapable of understanding. In one well-known American hospital the superintendent meets all new patients at a regular weekly meeting. He is introduced to each one. They are then gathered in the day room and he gives a five-minute talk about the hospital. This is group psychotherapy of the highest order.

At the Boston Dispensary there has been in existence for a number of years a so-called Thought Control Class. The class was formed and still remains under the leadership of a well-known internist who organized it as the result of his experience with a woman who could not walk but finally did so after intensive psychotherapy. This patient is still a member of the class. The group is made up of psychoneurotics who are diagnosed by exclusion. When no organic basis can be found for somatic complaints, the patient is referred to the Thought Control Class, and it is a significant fact that few patients will attend without urging. They insist that they are not mental cases. A physician is always in charge. He gives a short, simple, somewhat childlike, but always encouraging talk. The main portion of the time is taken up by the patients. Each one rises and gives her experience. Simple? Yes. Childish? Possibly, but he is dealing with people who are emotionally at an infantile level. Remember that this clinic is not conducted by a charlatan or quack but by a well-recognized internist who knows that a great many patients coming to him have no pathological basis for their complaints. He treats them on an emotional level and corrects their difficulties.

Group psychotherapy of this kind has a decided place in the mental hospital. Granted that its rationale cannot be demonstrated in a test tube or under the microscope and that it is purely empirical, it does improve the mental attitude of patients. All psychiatrists cannot do group therapy. It requires a special type of personality. I have seen the response in a group of four hundred patients who were assembled every day in the chapel for fifteen minutes before going to their work. A few songs, a few simple exercises, and an enthusiastic talk sent them away heads up and smiling. Why do we psychiatrists refuse to recognize the methods that are found so useful with armies, Rotary Clubs, and other adult organizations?

Nurses should be instructed in the technique of getting the patients on the ward together for a daily chat. One of the best reasons for doing this is the daily newspaper. At a regular time each evening everyone should be assembled in the day room. The nurse sits with them. She hands the paper to the first patient and asks him to read a particular article, announcing that everyone must listen closely because they will discuss it afterwards. The patient reads the article, which should not be too long, and the nurse calls upon certain patients to tell what they think about it. One half-hour each day can be spent profitably this way. It keeps the patients in touch with reality. If mental hospital nurses would stimulate more patients to do this kind of thing, we would have better psychiatric nursing. The sooner she looks upon herself as a teacher and leader the more rapidly will she really begin to do something for her patients.

The Radio. The installation throughout the hospital of a system of radio loud speakers which are controlled from a central point offers a means of dissemination of the spoken word to patients which may in time become a very important factor in suggestive therapeutics. The radio has become an essential part of our modern life and has influenced the thought of nations to an almost inconceivable degree. If radio suggestion is worth its tremendous cost to the manufacturer in increased sales, it must be a powerful suggestive factor to normal individuals. Is it not reasonable to suppose that radio suggestion can be utilized in the treatment of groups of psychotic patients? Special techniques and methods of putting out such suggestion will have to be formulated. There are many questions that will have to be answered by careful experimentation. The question as to how many hours a day a radio should operate, what kind of programs are calculated to give the best result, and what kind of music has the best therapeutic effect will require considerable study. While experience with normals constitutes a good point at which to begin, certainly some modification and elaboration will be necessary in order to achieve a maximum result with psychotic patients.

Out of a practical experience with a radio system certain principles have been evolved that should be mentioned. The management of broadcasting in a mental hospital must be such that patients feel they have some part in its management and some share in building its progress. If it is managed in a dictatorial fashion it will not accomplish the same purpose. Questionnaires concerning programs should be circulated among patients. When the patient feels that he can voice an opinion and ask for a particular program, he takes a greater interest in the radio. Many announcements are made during programs asking patients to write letters with suggestions in regard to changes or additions. I have known 100 letters to come from patients regarding a particular program. The technique used in ordinary radio broadcasting of offering prizes for the best letter containing suggestions is an excellent way of getting patients interested.

A radio system will not run itself. It must be the responsibility of one individual who has sufficient enthusiasm and interest to work out proper techniques. The logical individual is the musical director of the hospital. He should be a musician and have sufficient administrative ability to organize and plan special features. Patients may be used as announcers. It is an exceedingly valuable type of occupation for certain psychoses. Those who are verbal exhibitionists find working in the radio room exceedingly interesting and worth while. Such a system must be managed exactly like a commercial station if it is to do the maximum amount of good. Four to five hours' broadcasting from the hospital radio room will accomplish a great deal in the way of constructive therapy.

There are two types of advertising in the commercial world. The first is lengthy, costly, showy, and impressive. The other, which is used more frequently, is brief and to the point, and eventually makes an impression by its constant persistence and dogged determination. Both of these psychological approaches which are employed to influence groups can be used with the hospital radio. The first type is given in the form of playlets, talks, and musical programs. The second comes to the patient in the form of mental hygiene hints that are incorporated in the regular programs. Instead of using the ordinary commercial announcement, this time is taken by the hospital station for diversified hygienic tidbits. These hints include explanatory bits on occupational therapy, the psychoses, the various types of therapy, and other interesting items about the institution.

For patients to get the maximum effect from these planned programs, they must be urged to listen. The formal local programs should be given at a regular time. Nurses and attendants must accept the responsibility for having all of the patients on the ward in the space where the radio is and insisting that they listen. Patients should be urged to express their opinion of the program in writing. Frequent reports by head nurses and attendants are sent to the radio room in order that some check may be made as to the efficacy of the programs. If radio is to be used as a therapeutic measure every effort must be made to see that the patient takes the medicine, and to check the result.

What is the general effect upon the patients of this kind of group suggestion?

I. It improves the general morale of patients.

A. Lessens antagonism to hospital.

The moment the patient enters a mental hospital he transfers to the institution the antagonism that has existed between himself and society. Anything that will lessen this feeling is a useful adjunct to treatment. All patients cannot be interviewed by the superintendent but they can be reached collectively by means of a radio. Regular weekly talks by the head of the hospital are particularly appealing to the patient. Such a talk bears the stamp of authority and is listened to with respect by the majority of patients. For the admission wards, a series of four talks can be given. The first is a general orientation for the patient. Acquaint him with the institution, emphasizing the fact that he is in a hospital. Details such as the explanation of church services, letters, and similar bits of information are outlined. Many of these points have already been covered in the admission letter. But they should be repeated as many times and by as many people as possible. The second talk would deal with the methods of legal commitment. In our experience this is one of the most important talks of the series.

Patients are always in a state of confusion as to the legality of their commitment, and a clear exposition of the law governing these matters is received gratefully and does much to clarify the patient's mind. The third talk deals with methods of treatment. It tells about hydrotherapy, occupational therapy, physiotherapy, the medical service, etc. It attempts to orient the patient with regard to what treatment may be expected. The last talk is based purely on mental hygiene. Certain dogmatic statements must be made for the patient to think over. The conduct that will be expected of him while he is a member of the hospital group should be outlined in detail. Weekly talks are given by members of the medical staff, the nursing instructors, the occupational therapists, and members of the business departments. All take their turn at the microphone in order to fully acquaint the patients with what is going on in the hospital.

B. Disseminates information about the work of the hospital.

The mental hospital is a community. It is our purpose to try to get the patient to become a good citizen of the institution as a preliminary to his return to his own community. A good citizen takes an interest in something outside of himself and lends assistance and coöperation to society. A good patient will take an interest in the community in which he is, and the more he knows about what the departments are doing, the better hospital citizen he will be.

C. Makes patient feel that he is a part of the group.

These talks by members of the different departments are an indication that one is not alone in the hospital, that there are many other people in similar circumstances and that each one of these can, in their small way, help to rehabilitate themselves.

D. Keeps up the interest of the patient in the outside world.

We are constantly endeavoring to get patients to accept reality. The fact remains, and we cannot get away from it, that in a mental hospital the windows are barred, the doors are locked, and many rigid rules are enforced. All of this may be psychologically a contributing factor to the sense of isolation which a patient may feel after commitment. Before the days of radio, the only connection with the outside world was an occasional visit from a relative or an infrequent concert by philanthropic outsiders. Today there is hardly an important event that it is not possible to bring to the most disturbed ward in the hospital. Political events of state or national importance, such as a speech by the President of the United States, should interest any individual, and the fact that these events can be broadcast to wards is an emphatic declaration that they are no more isolated than their relatives who are listening to the same program in their homes.

II. It disseminates information about mental hygiene.

The mental hygiene organizations are doing much to educate lay groups about the cause and treatment of mental disease. What community group could benefit to a greater extent by such talks than our own patients? Radio lectures of 10 to 15 minutes' duration relative to mental diseases are well received by patients. They must be simply worded and given in an informal manner. One series would deal with the psychoses, telling simply but plainly what dementia praecox or general paresis is. Obviously the psychiatrist cannot pour out an avalanche of technicalities in this situation. He must use simple language if he is to reach his audience. A series of purely psychological talks dealing with such subjects as mental mechanisms, nervous exhaustion, sublimation, projection, etc., are a part of this educational program. The positive proof that patients do enjoy, benefit from, and appreciate this type of talk is manifested by their verbal comments and their letters.

RECREATION

The radio is almost a necessity for the majority of human beings in this country. It is a source of pleasure to many people. A mental hospital with all modern types of therapy, equipment, and installation is still a house of sighs and sorrows. Everything that can serve to alleviate any of this discontent should be utilized. Entertainment is therapeutic, but if we divorce it from its therapeutic side we still have assets in its utilization. Many hours a week are made more bearable to the patients of the hospital by listening to the baseball games. This one feature alone is serving a triple purpose. It is providing positive entertainment, it is emphatically socializing the patient's mind and interest, and it is bringing him back to reality.

SELF-EXPRESSION

A minority of patients in mental hospitals are musically talented and receive great satisfaction from expressing their ability before an audience. The mechanical fascination of a microphone makes even normal individuals tense. It calls for mental discipline and its demand is even more insistent than the eyes of an audience. Performing over the radio can become a therapeutic situation both for the patient performer and listeners. Broadcasting by patients is a part of the therapeutic benefit accomplished.

RACIAL PROGRAMS

Most mental hospitals have a large foreign population, many of whom speak the English language poorly or not at all. A thousand speeches in English would not equal one single sentence in their mother tongue to these individuals. A Polish folk song brings forth more reaction from a Slavic patient than would a symphonic poem.

SPECIAL PROGRAMS

Positive suggestion in getting patients to coöperate with a ward program of activity is valuable. Fifteen minutes before each meal broadcasts to all continued treatment wards give certain direct commands. "Wash your face, comb your hair, lace your shoes, get ready for lunch." Constant repetition of this in a monotonous voice may attract the attention of patients. Direct suggestion by radio to the pack room is worth a trial. The suggestion of sleep monotonously repeated should give satisfactory results. Would it be possible to think of the radio in terms of artificial hallucinations that would guide the patient along the lines of normal behavior? Patients are governed by auditory hallucinations in their conduct in spite of anything that may be said by those around them. A fantastic idea? Well, perhaps, but who knows? It has never yet been tried. There are many ways by which psychiatrists can utilize this modern mechanical device for purely psychotherapeutic purposes.

OTHER WAYS OF DISSEMINATING SUGGESTION

Inspection trips through the hospital. A group of newly admitted patients would derive a great deal of benefit from an inspection trip of the hospital. Five or six patients should be taken to the offices and shown how the letters are handled, how telephone calls are taken care of, how case records are prepared. They visit the library and a short talk is given by the librarian. The steward's office and the office where their money is kept are points of interest. A visit to the industrial rooms shows mattress making, furniture refinishing, and the many things that are carried on. They go to the kitchen, the engine room, the cow-barn, and any other place that will serve to give them a better understanding of what the hospital's problems are and how the organization is built around their particular needs.

MOVING PICTURES ON WARDS

The recent development of the 16-millimeter projector with sound makes it possible for the mental hospital to have a portable outfit by means of which patients can be shown suitably selected pictures directly on the wards. Excellent films are available, and an occasional picture for the closed wards and for those who are physically ill would be beneficial.

WARD SOCIAL EVENTS

The entertainment of one ward by another is a factor of great importance in bringing a normal life to our patients. We ask them to live a homosexual social existence and wonder that they are not satisfied with it. A women's ward giving a social event for a male ward surely cannot do very much harm if it is properly supervised. I am thoroughly aware of the administrative problems that it may bring up. But I believe that more of these small, informal group parties would be extremely beneficial to psychotic patients.

BIRTHDAY CARDS FOR PATIENTS

The date of birth of every patient who comes to the hospital is known. It would not be a particularly laborious clerical task to keep a record of these dates in a follow-up card system, and on the proper date send a greeting card to the patient with the compliments of the hospital. Such an attention would serve to build up a great deal of good will.

VISITING GROUPS FOR PATIENTS

The mental hospital has always been reluctant to permit the community to assist in the care of patients. In the general hospital the idea of such visiting groups is utilized to the very fullest extent and the hospital reaps a considerable benefit materially from this coöperation. I can see no reason why groups of philanthropic women and men cannot be organized from the community to visit patients who are in sufficiently good condition to make such visits of therapeutic value. This idea has been tried in mental hospitals, and particularly among those patients who are physically ill. A group of women from the community designated two of their number to visit certain wards of a mental hospital each week. The benefit to the patients in a therapeutic way was immeasurable. It is a plan that should be elaborated upon and carried much further. I am quite familiar with all arguments against it, but I maintain that it is a useful measure. The record of the lodge to which a male patient belongs could very well be kept by the hospital and a visiting committee from that particular order invited to visit these patients at regular intervals. The formation of lodges and clubs within the hospital population itself is an idea that has been tried in mental hospitals with success. A legally chartered organization of Campfire Girls was the means by which one hospital treated its younger women patients socially. The system of rewards and merits which are given for homely tasks is particularly efficient in handling a psychotic group of individuals.

GRADING PATIENTS

An attempt has been made to set up a grading system on a ward, with very excellent results. This plan divides the patients into groups according to behavior. Signs are placed on the wall, showing what an individual has to do to get into each group.

A. At home

B. Going home:
Works well
Reliable—on parole
New interests and new ideas
Old ideas forgotten

C. On Parole:
Works and plays well
Obeys rules
Getting new ideas and interests
Making the best of everything
Playing the game and coöperating in everything

D. First Class on the Ward:
Keeps neat and tidy
Works well and plays well
Learning to take things as they come
Beginning to forget old ideas
Learning to coöperate in everything

E. Second Class on Ward:
Works poorly and plays poorly
Careless of clothes
Satisfied to sit around and rest
Proud of own ideas and unwilling to listen to others
Not very coöperative

F. Third Class on Ward:
Little or no work or games
Silent or too talkative
Excitable and disturbed at times
No coöperation and no trying
Mute and resistive

A visible record is kept showing the names of the patients in each group. Relatives are fully as interested in watching this board as are the patients themselves. Perhaps an improvement on the idea would be an attempt to actually grade wards in a more formal manner and classify the patients on these wards in accordance with their type of behavior. If certain wards could be set aside for a certain kind of behavior, the requirements for remaining on this ward being clearly set forth in attractive signs, it would be a considerable incentive for patients to conform. One of the difficulties patients have is to work out in their own minds what kind of conduct constitutes normal conduct. If this could be better formalized and presented to the patient, it would be an inducement to correct his abnormal behavior.

In these and countless other ways the administrator sets up an organized effort to use group therapy and change the attitude of patients into normal channels. By the power of suggestion he constantly surrounds individuals with educational propaganda designed to keep them in touch with reality. Every mental hospital could well afford to attach to the staff a director of propaganda who would study and elaborate, for therapeutic application, the many mediums through which we are constantly receiving suggestion in our modern community life. This is group psychotherapy.

Chapter 8

OCCUPATIONAL AND INDUSTRIAL THERAPY

Occupation is one of the oldest forms of psychiatric therapy. It is mentioned by Hippocrates, and was an important part of the treatment carried on in the early Greek temples, the first sanatoria of which we have any record. In the old reports of American mental hospitals it is discussed at length, and much emphasis was placed on its benefit to the patient. Occupational therapy became a distinct profession following the World War. The large number of neuropsychiatric patients created a need for a more systematic and better conceived plan of work therapy for the psychotic veteran. At present occupational therapy has developed to the point where its representatives have become indispensable to many general, tubercular, orthopedic, and mental hospitals.

While there is little evidence that occupational therapy has a specific effect upon the psychoses, there is much evidence to show that it has considerable influence upon the personality of the patient. Concentration upon a difficult task creates an interest on the part of the patient. It compels his attention. Absorption in a piece of work is a substitute for the disorganized thoughts and ideas which are the manifestations of the psychosis. It establishes new enthusiasms, builds up an altruistic spirit, is a sedative for emotional unrest, gives courage instead of discouragement, and has a decidedly normalizing effect upon psychotic patients. Work is a part of reality—interest in it brings the patient back from his world of phantasy into contact with his surroundings. It is substitution therapy.

While mental hospitals have always utilized patients in their industrial activities, there has been a distinct line of demarcation between occupational and industrial therapy. The former has been primarily an application of the crafts, and trained therapists have not been greatly concerned with what should be the real goal of all occupational treatment—a useful industry that fits the patient to become a contributing member of the hospital or general community. A feeling has developed, not expressed but implied by attitudes on the part of many therapists, that industrial work is not occupational therapy. This is a narrow viewpoint and one which should be corrected by educational institutions which instruct occupational therapists. Any form of work is therapeutic and must be classified as such. But used as it has been in the past, it is reaching only a small number of patients, doing a minimum amount of good, and serving only a fractional part of its real usefulness. If the entire work program of the hospital could be organized around the idea of therapy, we should be using a valuable form of treatment in a more intelligent way.

There are two factors which must be taken into consideration when planning such a program. The first of these is the psychological needs of the patient. If work is to be real treatment it must be considered primarily from that point of view. The assignment of patients to industrial places cannot be a frantic scramble to get jobs filled because work has to be done. Prescriptions are as important in occupation as they are in drug therapy. A physician who would not think of asking a pharmacist to give some medicine to a patient for indigestion has no hesitation in requesting the occupational therapist to put a schizophrenic patient to work. In the application of any therapeutic procedure the psychiatrist must know a great deal about the emotional needs of the patient. For what is the employment to be prescribed? What does he hope to accomplish by it? What kind of work would best suit the needs of the patient? But in addition to his knowledge of the patient, the pyschiatrist must know something about the occupation which is being prescribed. If he believes that the needs of the patient will be best met by assigning him to the laundry, he should be reasonably familiar with the kind of occupation carried on there. To send a patient to the laundry and permit the head laundryman to use him where needed is to defeat the object of the prescription. It is not therapy but thoughtless placement.

The second factor which must always be taken into consideration in planning occupational therapy policies is the economic need of the hospital for the product of the patient's labor. We cannot evade the fact that patient labor is a necessity to the mental hospital. The institution could not carry on if it were not available. Light, heat, and power must be produced. Farming activities are essential for food. Patients and employees must be fed. Laundry facilities are vital to its existence. All of these departments depend upon the work of patients and most of them are on a production and time basis. Meals must be served at regular hours. Weeds will choke out plants unless promptly eliminated. Clothing must be washed when soiled. It would be prohibitive in cost to hire people to carry on these industries, but more than this, it would take from the psychiatrist one of his most important methods of treatment.

Are these two objects incompatible? Can the patient be the first consideration in prescribing occupational therapy and at the same time the economic requirements of the hospital be taken care of? It will be the purpose of this chapter to develop the thesis that both of these objects can be attained by a properly organized program of occupational therapy.

Organized, systematic work is better treatment than careless, haphazard occupation. Every administrator is familiar with the grotesque ways of working which many patients adopt when permitted to work out their own methods. This is an indictment of our training and supervision. The patient who is placed in a work environment where the activity is carried on in an orderly manner will respond better and derive more benefit than the one who is taken to the shop and permitted to do the work in his own way without instruction or training. There is one best way of doing handwork of any kind. The patient must be carefully trained by the supervisor in the technique of doing the work.

For instance, a mental hospital using a cafeteria food service had a great deal of difficulty with the organization of the tray room. The patients left their trays at a slide in the rear of the dining room. These trays were passed along a metal shelf, from one patient to another, each one removing a particular dish. The noise and confusion created an atmosphere in which it was difficult to get patients to work. The trays could not be handled fast enough and they jammed in the opening. The patients worked under great pressure. The breakage was high. It would take a considerable stretch of imagination to call work of this kind, performed in such an environment, occupational therapy. The thoughtful administrator knows it is not.

A moving belt was installed to carry the trays from the opening to the last man. The belt moved at a speed which permitted each patient sufficient leisure to remove his particular dish easily and quietly. Each man was carefully instructed in the exact motions to accomplish his part in an efficient manner.

The result was astounding. The room became one of the important therapeutic points in the hospital. The psychiatrist was able to assign convalescent patients to this task, and it became very popular. The belt took away all noise and confusion, and made the entire process an orderly procedure instead of a disorganized, haphazard plan of operation. And from the economic point of view, breakage was cut down 68 per cent and the number of men needed to do the work reduced by half.

In most mental hospitals little thought is given to the planning of a vegetable preparation room. The usual lay-out is a large area adjacent to the kitchen, containing a sink and many chairs or benches. Here women patients sit in the débris, carrying on the work of preparing vegetables with only the most perfunctory supervision. The result is dirt and filth, waste of vegetables, small production, and what is more important than all, the work is not only not beneficial to the patient but in some cases actually harmful. Careful thought and planning completely revolutionized the situation in one mental hospital and made of it a valuable therapeutic occupation. In considering the renovation, the principle of system and order was held as the important thing. And what would benefit the patient would increase production. Since the vegetable preparation room is a factory, those planning the new room turned to industry for their model. A receiving division was built where vegetables could be received and weighed, keeping the dust and dirt away from the finished product. A long, narrow, metal bench was installed on a fourteen-inch platform and fifteen women, in white uniforms and caps, were seated at the bench in comfortable work chairs. In front of each woman were three openings. The one at the left was rectangular and of a size to contain a pan of vegetables. Directly in front of her were two round openings. Into the one on the left she pushed the débris and into the one on the right she deposited the finished vegetable. Both of these openings had cylindrical chutes which led into buckets on the floor. The vegetable pans were exchanged as rapidly as emptied.

Here the transformation in the atmosphere of the room was striking. It immediately became a valuable occupation for the psychiatrist to prescribe. The same group of patients changed overnight from a quarreling, noisy group of psychotic patients to quiet, orderly, and industrious women. The therapeutic effect was nothing short of a miracle. The installation of a radio made a still further improvement in the environment and incidentally increased the number of vegetables handled. On the economic side, waste has been cut down because of the inspection of each patient's work and production has increased practically 100 per cent.

Who can say that such orderly occupations are not as therapeutic as the crafts. All that is needed is the goal of treatment and careful planning. And what has been accomplished in these departments can be done in every industrial division of the hospital. Each industry can be reorganized on the basis of the therapeutic needs of the patient. The industrial worker has never been seriously considered as an occupational therapist. Patients have been assigned to him for employment, but he has been given no information that would lead him to develop an interest in the patient as a sick human being. The workman sees himself as one who is hired to do a certain kind of work. The patient is a helper, and he feels no responsibility beyond getting a certain amount of work done. The attendant who takes a group of patients out to work on the farm interprets his position as that of a guard whose chief business is to prevent escapes. Rarely does he see himself as a teacher and instructor. There have been notable exceptions, but these have usually been workmen and attendants who have achieved this as a result of their own personal vision and initiative and not as a result of a planned administrative policy. Group occupation can be made a socializing process if thought is given to the organization of the work.

One of the most interesting examples of industrial therapy I have seen was worked out by the steward of a mental hospital. He had no thought of the therapeutic effect but was actuated by economic motives. But this illustrates the point that real treatment and production are compatible. A building was in the process of construction and a group of deteriorated patients were unloading bricks from a truck and placing them in a shed. The distance the bricks had to be carried was about forty feet. There was need for haste because the car would go on demurrage the next day. The work progressed at a snail-like pace. Each patient shuffled up to the truck, took two bricks, and shuffled back to the pile. The group was a disorganized mob. The steward stood it as long as he could and then took command of the situation. He organized the patients by placing them about two feet apart in a line from the truck to the pile. The first patient took two bricks from the truck, passed them to the next man, and so on down the line. When the method was learned, the bricks began to disappear from the truck like snow in the sun, and the speed with which that car was unloaded amazed even the man who organized it. And the effect upon the patients was remarkable. Each was dependent upon the other. Each one straightened up and slowly worked into a swinging rhythm, and the animation in their facial expressions indicated what the therapeutic effect was. The incident helped to impress upon me the fact that the needs of both hospital and patient can be met by proper work organization.

It is true that mechanics must have skill but it is equally true that skill alone will not be sufficient for the hospital which is interested in real occupational therapy. The personality of the workman is of equal importance. His ability to get along with patients and his willingness to accept the policy of the hospital that he must teach and instruct should always be taken into consideration when selecting employees. With such an attitude, the economic interests of the hospital are better taken care of. A carpenter who can train three or four patients to do simple carpentry and make repairs under his supervision contributes more to the patients and increases his production over that of the man who sees in the patient assigned to his department a helper to fetch and carry for him. If occupational therapy is to be the factor in the hospital that it should be, the development must be along these lines.

Administrative attempts to reorganize the occupational program along these lines will meet with many discouragements through the traditional attitudes on the part of both psychiatrists and workmen. The psychiatrist must assume the responsibility for knowing more about the work of the hospital, and he tends to evade this. The workmen and other employees have thought of patients as helpers so long that they change slowly. But quiet, persistent pressure from the administration will slowly but surely change the entire industrial atmosphere into a situation where every man and woman is a therapist.

One of the most important factors in effecting this change is the training and understanding of the chief occupational therapist. Her position is a strategic one. She is the individual who carries on the liaison between the various departments. It is she who furnishes inspiration and who stimulates each individual to carry out the policies. She introduces the patient to the job, checks on his work, and in frequent consultation with psychiatrist and employee brings to each the difficulties and perplexities of the other. Upon her rests the responsibility of instructing nurses and attendants, industrial workers and department heads. She keeps records of the work of the patients and the grades given them by industrial therapists, and prepares statistics showing progress. She becomes one of the most important individuals in the organization. But it should be pointed out that in all this her department must have the complete support and active assistance of the administrator and his professional and lay councils. Without it she can do nothing. Encouragement, guidance, and leadership are essential if she is to carry out such policies. The program will succeed or fail in proportion to her ability to weld the entire group together. She will be to industrial therapy what the director of nursing is to the ward service.

The occupational therapist who follows out the traditions of her training and sees herself only as a teacher of a class in craftwork will be of little value in a program of this kind. Her vision will have to go far beyond such a narrow viewpoint. The crafts have a place in the scheme, but are only introductory to a broader training. She must have good grounding in craft work but will use it as a means to an end rather than as an end in itself.

A man whose wife had made an excellent recovery called at the hospital after her return home to discuss with the psychiatrist certain phases of the illness. He was very laudatory of the efforts of the hospital, but during the course of conversation burst out with this illuminating comment, "Why didn't you teach my wife to do something besides crocheting? She wants to sit all day and do nothing else." The hospital may have given her a hobby but it did not teach her to carry her home responsibilities. It did not recognize that crafts must be the introduction and not the end.

A broader conception of the place of occupational therapy has not yet been completely adopted by occupational leaders. The essence of the formal training they receive is in craft work. But a number of schools where therapists are educated have accepted the broader viewpoint. Practical training in psychiatric hospitals during the undergraduate period permits students to acquire a better understanding of the needs of the patient. The chief occupational therapist must have not only technical training and the proper conception of her contribution but also the personality traits that make her a leader in the organization. Her education and general cultural background must inspire the respect of other professional members of the group. She must make her own place in the organization, and no amount of authority or administrative support will make up for a deficiency in these characteristics.

As has been pointed out, the psychiatrist, in his application of this occupational scheme, must know the job as well as the patient. He must be familiar with the therapeutics of the medicine if he is to prescribe it intelligently. Turning to industry for guidance along this line, we find that a job analysis is the first step of the personnel manager to fit the worker to the job.

Psychiatrists and supervisors probably have a general idea of the requirements of many industrial positions in the hospital. Most of this information has been accumulated in a vague way but it lacks definiteness and clarity. It is the duty of the occupational therapist to gather these ideas from all quarters and bring them into coherence and order for the use of those who are applying occupational therapy.

No one can sit in an office and out of thin air obtain a job analysis. Such an analysis requires an actual first-hand study of the operation, and to do this the therapist must actually be in the industry for a sufficient time to grasp some idea of its processes as they affect the patient.

Here we meet our first resistant attitude. The therapist who goes into the laundry to study its processes may find herself viewed with suspicion by the laundry workers. They look upon her as a spy who is gathering information about them for the administrator. For this reason, any attempt to make such an analysis must always be preceded by a period of education which sets forth the object of the study. This can come only from the administration. The executive who wishes to make an industrial survey will find it worth while to call together all the workers in the department where the study is to be made and to explain to them in simple, non-technical language the reason for the analysis. Coöperation will be better if workers know the reasons for the study.

As an example of the difficulties in achieving results when knowledge is not made available to those involved, the following is constructive: A hospital had two barns in close proximity to each other. One housed a small herd of cattle with contagious abortion, which was gradually being eliminated, and the other a clean herd. A great deal of difficulty was experienced in getting employees to observe certain precautions when passing from one barn to the other. Rules were posted, employees were reprimanded and occasionally discharged, but the carelessness continued. Finally all barn employees and patients were brought to the laboratory and the pathologist demonstrated to them the responsible bacillus, the manner of its transmission, and how it affected the milk. The trouble was corrected. Both employees and patients understood why such precautions were necessary. They had previously interpreted these precautionary measures as a ritual thrust upon them by a tyrannical administration.

And so with industrial workers. It is a constant wonder to me why we get as good coöperation as we do, considering the mystery that surrounds so many of our rules and regulations. Employees are usually willing to play the game enthusiastically if they know how and why. They should be taught the rules before being asked to play. And having been educated as to the reason for such an analysis and survey, those who cannot or will not understand and coöperate should be eliminated from the organization. One scoffing, skeptical employee will sour the whole group and the administrator will find himself against a stone wall of indifference.

Preliminary to the detailed job analysis a complete classification of patient industrial positions should be made. This should cover every department of the hospital and should give the kind of work and the sex and number of patients required.

After this classification has been worked out by the occupational therapist she proceeds to establish a minimum quota of workers for each division of the industry. This quota is assigned on the basis of her job analysis and in conference with the department head and the employee who is immediately in charge of the unit.

The following scheme for making an occupational analysis is offered as an example:

JOB ANALYSIS

Hospital Department
Department Head

Division
Division Head

Attitude of Department Head. Give your impression of his attitude towards the policy of utilizing his industry for treatment. Is he willing to change or does he resist interference with the routine? Does he thoroughly understand the motive back of the plan?

Attitude of Division Head. The individual who is in direct charge of the employees in the division is important, and every attempt should be made to show him how his own responsibilities can be more efficiently carried out. Give your impression of his attitude.

Attitude of Industrial Therapist. This is the employee who is in charge of a unit of the division and who comes directly in contact with the patient. Does he instruct the patients in work technique? Is his personality one that attracts others? Does he understand the importance of the patient? Is he teachable? Give your impression of the future possibility of development along the lines indicated.

Description of Work. Note whether it is performed sitting or standing, alone or in company with others, what degree of concentration is needed, whether strength is required. Give a detailed description of the exact process.

Environment. A description of the place where the work is carried on should include cleanliness, sanitation, equipment, ventilation, lighting, warmth, rest-rooms, pressure of production, instruction given, rest periods, and general efficiency of the group. Give an impression of the atmosphere of the conditions under which the work is done, and always include personalities as a part of the environment.

Supervision. Some work cannot be performed under close supervision. Give the degree of supervision—constant, intermittent, slight, none. Note whether department is locked or whether more freedom must be given because of the nature of the work.

Industrial Hazards. Note all the hazards to which the patient will be exposed. Tripping and falling, handling heavy objects (overstrain), defective structures, defective guards for machinery, defective hand tools, insufficient tools and equipment, electrical hazards, crowded conditions, carelessness, ignorance, lack of coöperation.

Requirements of the Job. Physical: what is needed in the physical make-up of the patient? Strength, height, weight, physical disability.

Psychological: Give the necessary mental qualifications. Alertness, intelligence, blocking, retardation, day-dreaming.

Social: Give your impression of the social qualities needed for the work.

Working Hours. The number of hours that patients work is very important. Note whether substitutions are possible in order to make shorter hours for particular patients.

Uniforms Worn. A uniform is sometimes a valuable aid in attracting the attention of a patient to a particular job.

All information should be summed up in an impressionistic picture of the occupation which will give the psychiatrist the information he needs to understand what the patient is to do.

To illustrate the working of this scheme, a finished analysis made in the laundry of a mental hospital is given.

JOB ANALYSIS, *State Hospital*

Department—Steward; *Division*—Laundry; *Division Head* —John Doe; *Industrial Therapist*—James Doe.

Unit of Division: Flatwork Ironer

Attitude of Department Head. The head of this department has been in his present position fifteen years. He has seen many innovations tried, some good and some bad. He thoroughly understands the fact that the primary business of the hospital is to treat patients and he recognizes his own responsibility in this object. He points out that the laundry is one of the vital industries of the hospital. It must go on, and there will always be great pressure for production. The general attitude of the steward is understanding. He will be sympathetic and give real coöperation.

Attitude of Division Head. The present head has held his position for the past three years. While primarily trained as an industrial foreman, his intelligence and ability to organize the flow of work plus the technical training given him by his immediate superior have made him a very efficient laundryman. His attitude towards the patients is kindly and humane. He is ready to accept guidance in handling them and appreciates the argument that the more carefully the patient is selected and the better he is trained, the more efficient will be both treatment and output.

Attitude of Industrial Therapist. The individual in charge of the flatwork ironer is a young man who has been in his present position four years. He is pleasant and agreeable, and kind to patients, but he does not make any persistent attempt to train them. He is apt to do the work himself rather than take the slower way of instructing the patient. He is coöperative within his capacity, but only time and an actual demonstration will get him to the point where he appreciates what it is all about. He is teachable within limits.

Description of Work. The work consists of two parts, feeding flat pieces of linen into the ironer and removing them from the opposite end. It may be carried on either sitting or standing. Stools are provided. The large pieces, such as sheets and table cloths, are handled by two workers. The small pieces, such as towels, are handled by one.

Environment. The laundry is a hot, dark, dreary place to work. It is particularly disagreeable on cold, damp days. This particular work is not pleasant. In spite of the fact that the ironer is hooded and equipped with ventilating fans, it is not a pleasant job. The pressure of work is continuous but not too fatiguing.

The laundry is well organized and the general spirit of cooperation is excellent. But the volume of work is too heavy for the equipment and the result of this is that there is great pressure, particularly on the wash wheels.

Supervision. The doors of the laundry are locked, and closed ward patients can be assigned. The immediate supervision of the ironer is intermittent. One employee has the responsibility of the ironer and the process of "shaking out," but the two operations are carried on in close proximity to each other. Supervision, on the whole, is good. Instruction can be improved.

INDUSTRIAL HAZARDS

There are no special hazards created by the machine itself. It is so guarded that an accident cannot occur. But the hot, steamy atmosphere is a decided hazard. Going from the temperature of the laundry to the colder air outside may set up respiratory conditions, unless patients are protected by warm outer clothing.

REQUIREMENTS

Physical. Good physical condition is essential. Most of the work is done standing. Varicose veins, oedema of the feet, fallen arches, and limited use of one or both arms and legs are physical contra-indications.

Psychological. Patient should have ability to concentrate on simple routine movements. A fair degree of mental alertness is required. Pressure of work tends to correct slight degrees of blocking and day-dreaming.

Social. The necessity for working directly with another patient and indirectly in a large group demands some ability on the part of the patient to get along with others.

Working Hours. Patients are brought to their work at 8:00 A.M. They leave at 11:30, return at 1:30 P.M., and are through at 4:30. It is possible to have a morning and afternoon group trained.

Uniforms. No uniforms are worn but it is recommended that white shirts and trousers be issued to patient workers because of coolness and sanitary considerations.

Summary. This is an excellent place for certain types of patients. In spite of the fact that the work is heavy and is constantly pressing and the machinery is both antiquated and inadequate in capacity and convenience, the spirit of the employed group and the excellent quality of leadership make it an excellent place for the assignment of suitable patients. Those who work there show a loyalty to their jobs that reflects credit upon the employees. It can easily be developed into a real therapeutic occupational center.

Psychiatrist's Comment. This is a suitable occupation for patients who are able to make a fairly good institutional adjustment. It is sedative, has a certain social value, and requires a fair degree of concentration. It is habit training because of the constant repetition of the same movements. Mental defectives with an I.Q. of 50-60, hebephrenics who are not too deteriorated, paretics who do not show too much incoördination, and slightly deteriorated alcoholics would do well in this occupation.

Having a complete job analysis of every industry in the hospital, the psychiatrist can have no excuse for not knowing what he is prescribing. The occupational therapist then turns her attention to the task for acquiring special knowledge about the patient for the use of the physician. A careful and complete industrial history of each new patient is taken by the therapist. The statistical data are obtained from the psychiatric record, but as much as possible is secured from the patient. The following outline is used:

INDUSTRIAL HISTORY

Name	Diagnosis
Date of Birth	Date of Admission
Nationality	Intelligence Quotient
Language Spoken	Physical Condition
Education	Height Weight

Industrial Experience. Get a detailed account of the types of work that patient has performed. Places are of no importance. Avoid general statements like, "worked in shoe factory." What did he do in the shoe factory? Get exact description of the work performed. What is the patient's reaction to the different kinds of work in which he has been engaged?

Recreational Interests. Has he been an athlete? If so, record the special kind of activity in which he was interested. Is he musical? Give details. Record clubs and organizations to which he has belonged and get his reaction to each.

Has he any hobbies? If so, how serious is his interest in them?

Is he a collector? Get full details.

SPECIAL TALENTS

Has he any special talents? If so, what are they?

INFORMATION TO BE SECURED FROM NURSE

Can he get along with others?
Does he follow directions?
Can he be taught to work?
Is he industrious?
Does he show courtesy to others?

Has he initiative?
Is he resourceful?
Has he any mechanical skill?
Is he neat and orderly in his work?
Is he punctual?
Can he be trusted?
Is he able to accept any responsibility?

This information is recorded on a 7 x 9 card, buff for men and blue for women. The file is kept in the service office of the occupational therapist and is available when the psychiatrist and aide are assigning patients to occupation.

In formulating an occupational program the administrator will find it of great assistance to work out a comprehensive scheme of responsibility which can be a part of the hospital standard practice.

The following outline is used for students in a mental hospital where this idea of occupational therapy prevails:

PROGRAM FOR OCCUPATIONAL THERAPY, *State Hospital*

In any plan leading to the application of occupational therapy to a large group of mental patients, there are three main types to be considered. They are given in the order of importance.

A. *Newly Admitted Patients*

B. *Continued Treatment Group*
  a. Convalescent
  b. Semi-Disturbed
  c. Disturbed
  d. Senile

C. *Medical and Surgical Patients*
  a. General Medical Wards
  b. Special Groups
    1. Cardiac
    2. Surgical
    3. Orthopedic
    4. Neurological
    5. Tubercular

The relationship between occupational therapist and nurse has always been a difficult one. Each has refrained from stepping over into the territory of the other. This attitude, which has insisted upon a sharply drawn line of demarcation, has resulted many times in a no-man's land where the patient is lost. The latter sits day-dreaming while the nurse waits for the therapist to come and give him some work. The occupational worker has a group of disheveled individuals in her class. She does nothing about the matter because it is clearly the business of the nurse to see that the patients are properly dressed. The patient suffers while the two professions stand off debating their responsibilities.

In an attempt to outline the place of both nurse and therapist in an occupational program, we find great difficulty in fixing the exact point where the nurse leaves off and the therapist begins. We talk glibly about coöperation between the two, but real team-work is seldom the case.

I believe that a certain phase of occupational therapy is a direct division of psychiatric nursing. If this is true, the nurse bears the full responsibility for its application to the patient and the therapist acts as a technical adviser. Hers is primarily a teaching function.

With this division in mind we may separate occupational therapy into two parts:

A. Projects for which the nurse is responsible.
B. Projects for which the occupational therapist is responsible.

Projects which come under the direction of the nurse are all introductory to the work of the therapist. They include habit training, ward housekeeping, and ward classes in which simple occupation is carried on.

Occupation habit training is as essential as personal habit training. The patient has lost the desire to carry on useful employment. He must be stimulated and urged to adopt again habits of industry. Such training must begin early in his hospital residence and must be carried on constantly with the goal of industrial adjustment ever in mind. The place of the therapist in this ward training is to advise and suggest to the nurse the kind of occupation for which the patient seems best suited.

The nurse should have access to the industrial history of the patient and should be guided by the psychiatrist in applying occupational therapy. She is a vital factor in the industrial scheme. She can help or hinder the progress of the patient. She assists by urging him to get interested in an occupation, by encouraging him to continue, and by promptly suggesting his transfer to the pre-industrial shop or to hospital industry. There is a constant temptation for nurses to keep an efficient patient on the ward, at times to his own detriment. Administrators must set up such checks as will enable the psychiatrist to know whether she is doing her part. There are many subtle ways by which a nurse can create a desire on the part of the patient to remain on the ward. I have known nurses and attendants to suggest to a patient that a certain occupation would make a "sissy" of him.

The nurse is a vital part of the occupational program of the hospital and she cannot evade her responsibility by turning it over to the occupational therapist. Occupation is as much a part of psychiatric nursing as any other procedure, and the nurse who is not thoroughly trained in the simple forms is not a good psychiatric nurse.

She is also responsible for certain physical and recreational activities which are confined to the ward. Calisthenics and walking either out-of-doors or on the ward are part of her ministrations. In the field of recreation, ward games, group singing and reading, ward parties, and entertainments are included in psychiatric nursing and must be carried on by the nurse.

Projects that are the direct responsibility of the occupational therapist are pre-vocational shop work and industrial therapy. The only contribution the nurse makes to these is her encouragement and support of the patient. A patient may be sent directly from ward occupation to an industrial department. But in many cases further training and preparation will be needed before he is ready for hospital industry. This need is met by pre-vocational instruction. When the stage is reached where actual pre-vocational instruction should begin, the occupational therapist assumes for the first time full and complete charge of the treatment. The pre-vocational classes should be preparatory to the graduation of the patient directly into the industrial department. If it is decided that a woman might become a power-machine operator in the sewing room, she should be taught to operate a small power-machine in the class. If a woman is to be assigned to an ironing board in the laundry, she is taught to iron. If a man is to be given work that calls for handling tools, he must acquire manual dexterity in the class. Graduated work is the key-note of real occupational therapy—working from the simple to the complex. The patient may remain at any stage of this progression for an indefinite period of time but always the goal of hospital or outside industry is ahead. While no production is demanded of the pre-vocational shop except in numbers of patients who graduate, much useful hospital work is done. The same thing is true of ward occupation. The production of useless articles or articles which cannot be used in the hospital is not good therapy, except in certain special cases. Always the thought of what the patient is to do when he leaves the hospital must be kept in mind. Anything that will make him more efficient is good therapy. The shop offers an excellent opportunity for the study and analysis of occupations. It is the point at which much valuable information may be obtained about both patient and work. It is the favorable place for carrying on research projects. The entire question of fatigue should be studied carefully. Posture while working has not received the attention it deserves. There is a great need for work in colors and occupational tests. All of this research can be carried on in the pre-vocational shop.

In the physical field the therapist has no responsibility except in special cases. Many hospitals have physical directors, and there is unquestionably a place for such a technician in every mental hospital. But the time of this individual would be spent to better advantage if he devoted it to teaching, instructing, and encouraging nurses and attendants to work with patients along these lines rather than to take away from them a nursing function.

And finally the patient is assigned to a particular place which seems to meet his needs. He is taken to the department by the occupational therapist. She delivers the psychiatrist's prescription, introduces the patient to both division head and industrial therapist, and sees that he is properly initiated into his job. And his further progress will depend upon the understanding of the industrial employee as to his proper place in the therapeutic scheme.

The following set of instructions for industrial workers was issued for their guidance and help in appreciating the real purpose of occupation:

Instructions for Industrial Therapists. The employee who can instruct and intelligently supervise several patients, and by doing so assist them in the recovery of their mental health, is of more value to this hospital than the one who has the attitude of a boss. It is not good treatment to expect patients to do competent work without proper instruction and supervision. But it is excellent therapy to carefully train them and then hold them to a high level of performance. A certain amount of responsibility is good for mental patients, but it must be within the limit of their capacity. They cannot be held to the same measure of responsibility as an employee.

Physicians assign patients to an occupation on the basis of what the patient needs. It is not for the industrial therapist to question his judgment. And if, in the opinion of the psychiatrist, the work should be changed and the patient placed in another department, the industrial worker has no right to question such a decision. Too often in the past patients have been retained in departments to their detriment because it was thought that the work they were doing was indispensable. If a patient is re-assigned by the physician, another must be trained.

Patients sent to a particular industry may not be returned to the ward without the permission of the psychiatrist. The only exception to this would be an emergency. And when getting the permission to leave the patient on his ward, the industrial therapist will be required to give the reasons why he does not believe the work will benefit the patient. At least three days' trial should be given before finally deciding that he cannot be taught to do the work required.

The industrial worker in this hospital is employed as a teacher and supervisor of patients. They are known as industrial therapists. They make a greater contribution to both hospital and patient in these capacities than they can by only doing work. Good teachers are active among their patients, encouraging the laggards, stimulating the dull and depressed, and holding back the excitable and disturbed.

Patients should not be driven. Regular rest periods are essential and ten minutes out of each hour should be devoted to relaxation. The point at which fatigue shows itself is reached sooner than with normals. The symptoms are increased irritability, lack of attention, greater excitement, flushed face, and increased pulse rate. These signs should be watched for constantly.

Every industrial therapist is held responsible for the patients during the entire period of work. This means that he must hold each patient to a fair standard of conduct, prevent work being carried on in a peculiar way, discourage his delusions, and try to gain his good will.

Every industrial therapist must report daily on the form provided the names of the patients working in each period, the time they report, and the quality of work each one is doing. The grading will be done according to the following plan:

A. Excellent worker, behavior good. Can carry some responsibility.
B. Good worker under direction. Behavior good. Industrious.
C. Fair worker. Must be told what to do. Behavior fair.
D. Poor worker. Not troublesome. Kept on trial. May improve.
E. Behavior poor. Will not work. Cannot follow directions. Will probably not improve.

These policies govern all industrial work in this hospital. Department heads will be held responsible for the selection and retention of people who can carry them out. They are responsible for the attitude and spirit of coöperation of department personnel.

Division of Responsibility for Occupation. One may fix the responsibilities of the several groups concerned in this occupational scheme as follows:

A. *Psychiatrist*

1. To assign the patient to the work on the basis of his needs.

2. To know the results of his occupational prescriptions.
3. To guide, stimulate, and teach all employees who direct the working of patients.
4. To keep in close relationship with department heads and industrial activities and know exactly what he is prescribing.
5. To instruct and guide all those who are working with him as to what he is trying to accomplish.

B. *Nurse*

1. To train patients for advancement into hospital industry under the guidance and leadership of the occupational therapist.
2. To organize and carry on ward occupational classes as a preparatory step towards pre-vocational training.
3. To coöperate with industrial therapists by constantly impressing upon patients that work is curative.
4. To have patients properly dressed and ready for work at the appointed time and at the proper place.
5. To constantly promote patients from ward work to outside industry.

C. *Occupational Therapist*

1. To secure such information about both patient and industry as is needed by the psychiatrist for proper placement.
2. To train patients in the pre-vocational shop for hospital industry.
3. To introduce the patient to the job after the assignment is made by the physician.
4. To give the industrial therapist all the information available about the patient for the purpose of aiding him in carrying out his responsibility.
5. To act in a liaison capacity between the psychiatrist and other departments.

D. *Department Head*

1. To keep in close touch with psychiatrists; weekly conferences are desirable.
2. To maintain a high degree of supervision and instruction of patients among his employee group.

3. To keep before them the goal of curing patients rather than getting work done.
4. To judge their usefulness upon their ability to supervise patients rather than upon their capacity to do the work themselves.
5. To see that prompt and accurate reports of the work of patients are made daily.

E. *Industrial Therapist*

1. To learn everything possible about the patient and what the physician hopes to accomplish.
2. To be interested in the patient as a human being and not exclusively as a worker.
3. To teach, guide, and supervise the work of the patient both as to quality and quantity.
4. To make an accurate daily report on the patient to the psychiatrist.

We have in occupational therapy a powerful therapeutic weapon for the treatment of psychotic patients. But it is not sufficient to place a force that can be applied to all patients exclusively in the hands of a small number of professional therapists. At best they can reach only a few patients. The important thing is to create throughout the hospital an atmosphere of industry and to make occupation an activity that is approved by the patient group. This can only be accomplished by extending the responsibility of patient occupation to every employee of the institution. The goal of this essential activity should be revised. Emphasis on patient productivity as such should be minimized and replaced on the therapeutic effect which the patient may derive from such work.

Chapter 9

THE CONTRIBUTION OF SOCIAL WORK

SOCIAL work, as an integral part of medicine and psychiatry, is of recent origin. But the principles and practices of modern case work have a background of great antiquity. From time immemorial philanthropically minded men and women have worked assiduously to correct environmental conditions that apparently played a part in the causation of illness, poverty, and crime. Out of their efforts grew modern social service.

The organization of this work into a recognized profession began a few years ago and is still in process. Professionalization was an inevitable accompaniment of certain changes of attitude and thought in the medical group. With the development of instruments of precision and laboratory tests for pathological conditions, there came a determined attempt to place medical practice upon the foundation of an exact science. The social aspects of disease received little attention. It was a complete reversal of the attitude of the old-time general practitioner, who was short on science but long on social sense. From the ignorant physicians and barber-surgeons of the Middle Ages, the medical fraternity has grown into a group of highly specialized individuals. Medical practice has become a coöperative enterprise. No longer is the physician the only one who is interested in matters of health and disease. Many subsidiary groups have come into being, to concern themselves with the problems of public health. It was out of this period of evolution that medical social service emerged as a profession, and it has become an increasingly important adjunct to modern hospital practice. The fact that physicians have generally accepted this new division of the health army is a hopeful sign that they are again becoming aware of the social significance of disease. They are thinking of the patient in terms of the whole organism. The psychosomatic relationship is receiving much consideration from thoughtful physicians.

There is a general agreement that diagnostic efforts must be centered around the physical, psychological, and social aspects of the patient if disease is to be really understood, and there are many indications that this interest will continue and increase.

A number of factors have had a powerful influence on the rapid growth of social work in psychiatry. The contributions of Freud, which emphasized an individualistic psychology, stimulated a change of attitude towards the new profession. It is not the purpose of the writer to debate or even discuss the merits of psychoanalysis. Many administrators are antagonistic towards the whole concept. The older ones have lived through the rise and fall of many enthusiasms. But it can be said to those who see no virtue in the hypothesis of Freud and his disciples that until some other school of thought offers a better approach to the problems of psychiatry, it cannot be entirely rejected. Mere negativistic resistance gets us nowhere. Progressive psychiatrists are not content with mere descriptive psychiatry. They see a distinct relationship between the psychoses and community and family situations. The social worker is an invaluable aid in tracing out the ramifications of these points of contact.

A further impetus was given to social work by the amazing development of the mental hygiene movement which began in 1912. The principle upon which this crusade was founded was the need for correction in the hospital environment of the psychotic patient. But it was soon realized that the social situation in the family and community was equally important, if the psychosis were to be really understood. And when this fact emerged from the confusion that marked the beginning of the movement, the social worker was the one to whom the psychiatrist turned for assistance. She advanced to a position of greater responsibility in the psychiatric team.

Finally the development of the Child Guidance Clinic brought forth well-trained psychiatric social workers who were capable of treating members of the family while the psychiatrist worked with the patient. And it was in this setting that social service became an actual department of psychiatry. The worker, for the first time, was given an opportunity to do more than gather factual material about the physical environment of the patient. She became a social therapist. She not only manipulated the physical environment but she endeavored to reëducate those personalities with whom the patient came into contact and who had the most effect upon him. She became indispensable to the child psychiatrist.

The hospital accepted psychiatric social service early. But it is doubtful whether all administrators have followed the rapid changes of psychiatry in its recognition of the social worker's place in the therapeutic scheme. They have been slow to accept the changing concepts of mental disease. Dynamic psychiatry, with its emphasis upon the study of the emotional life of the individual, finds many difficulties in a hospital atmosphere. The personal prejudices of executives and the limitations of its application to the psychotic have all tended to keep hospital psychiatry on a descriptive level. The importance given to social service by the superintendent is some indication of the acceptance of dynamic psychiatry by the professional staff. The type of social case work demanded by the institution is also an index of an interest in therapy rather than mere diagnostic labeling of patients.

Social service began to function in mental hospitals largely as a result of the desire to supervise patients on temporary absence. There was little idea of therapy. The social worker was an investigator and parole officer who gathered together the facts regarding the environment of the patient at the time of his admission or evaluated the probable influence of the home situation upon him when he was released. Her contribution was descriptive and factual, but without any attempt to interpret these facts in terms of social treatment. She was not supposed to have any knowledge of psychiatric mechanisms. But the situation has changed. More training and greater psychiatric knowledge and experience are needed by the worker to carry her part of the closer relationship. The collaboration of psychiatrist and social worker results in a therapeutic program which is better balanced than is possible when each works alone. She has been taught to understand the psychiatric implications in family situations. She appreciates the mechanisms that prevent harmony and can take steps to change these mechanisms. She works with the members of the family, seeking to change their attitudes, while the psychiatrist endeavors to correct the behavior of the patient.

There were three phases of responsibility in our earlier conception of social service:

A. AFTER CARE

This included the regular and systematic visiting of patients on parole from the hospital and those who were in boarding homes.

B. MEDICAL HISTORIES

Securing data concerning the medical history of the patient was an important responsibility of the social worker.

C. INVESTIGATIONS

This included special investigations in the case of new patients, the consideration of applications for boarding, and inquiry into the family situation before the patient was discharged.

While this broad division of social service remains practically the same, elaboration of technique has made great progress, evidenced by the report of the Committee on Mental Hospitals of the American Association of Psychiatric Social Workers, published in 1934.[26] The splendid compilation of essentials of psychiatric social service technique in mental hospitals and mental hygiene clinics attached to mental hospitals prepared by this Committee is so comprehensive and important that I am taking the liberty of including it in this book.

THE COMPILATION

OF

ESSENTIALS OF PSYCHIATRIC SOCIAL SERVICE TECHNIQUE

IN

MENTAL HOSPITALS AND MENTAL HYGIENE CLINICS

ATTACHED TO MENTAL HOSPITALS

I. SOCIAL SERVICE PROCESSES OUTLINED:

A. Policy of intake.

B. A compilation of social history.

C. A summary of the complete record for a particular purpose.

D. A critical study of a record where intensive social service treatment is being carried on by analyzing:

1. Factors contributing to both the patient's difficulties and possibilities for his readjustment:
    a. Personality traits in childhood, adolescence, and adulthood in relation to:
        1. Patient himself
        2. The family group.
        3. Others.
    b. Physical health throughout life of
        1. Patient
        2. Family group.
    c. Mental health through life of
        1. Patient
        2. Family group.
    d. Environmental influences—intellectual, social, economic, recreational, occupational, religious or ethical, racial.
2. Patient's verbalization of situation, his recognition of reality and his solution.
3. Plans for social service treatment for both patient and family regarding:
    a. Modification of attitudes and environmental manipulation:
        1. In meeting immediate need of patient as he sees it.
        2. For new and continued use of interested individuals, determined by:
            a. Interviewee's attitudes, needs and possibilities for reciprocal planning.
            b. Attitudes between interested individuals and patient.
            c. Attitudes of interested individuals toward agency or worker.
        3. By use of community facilities:
            a. In anticipating community misconceptions.

- *b.* In application of same technique to agencies as to clients.
- *c.* Through the selection and services of agencies.

b. Growth of patient's understanding to activate:
- *1.* Discussion of difficulties with a view to giving emotional relief.
- *2.* Stimulation of new interests.
- *3.* Social participation.
- *4.* Development of socially acceptable habits.

4. Considerations limiting:
- a. Amount of scientific knowledge.
- b. Resources.
- c. Theory and practice.
- d. The development of the patient and his potentialities for different levels of adjustment.

5. Psychiatrist's and social worker's rôle:
- a. Service of psychiatrist.
- b. Organization and functions of the agency.
- c. Type of case.

E. Case conference.

F. Treatment by:
- 1. Environmental manipulation.
- 2. Changing attitudes by:
  - a. Redirecting emotional ties and encouraging the development of new ties.
  - b. Developing understanding.
  - c. Re-education.

G. Evaluation of Treatment.

II. SOCIAL SERVICE METHODS OUTLINED:

A. Consideration of conditioning influences in contact:
- 1. Agency represented by worker:
  - a. Administrative problems
    - *1.* Financial.
    - *2.* Facilities.
      - *a.* Hospital acceptance of acute or chronic cases or both.
      - *b.* Clinic acceptance for diagnosis or treatment, or both.

3. Staff personnel:
   a. Number (adequate for agency service).
   b. Training and experience.
   c. Personalities.
   d. Interrelationships.
   e. Security in permanency of positions.

b. Reciprocal attitude determining acceptance of agency by community.

c. Policy of intake:
   1. Function of agency—type of work done:
      a. Institutional, clinic or both.
      b. Mentally ill, problems of emotional maladjustment or both.
      c. Selection of cases limited by:
         (1) Legal restriction.
         (2) Residence.
         (3) Age.
         (4) Advisory service.
         (5) Source of referral.
            (a) Explanation of agency to prepare interviewee.
            (b) Contact of previous social worker with interviewee.
   2. Possibilities for treatment dependent upon interviewee's
      a. Recognition of a problem.
      b. Dissatisfaction with the present adjustment.
      c. Recognition of need for treatment.
      d. Expectation of results of treatment.
      e. Partial acceptance of own responsibility for problem.
      f. Willingness to assume personal responsibility for treatment.
      g. Potential adjustability.
      h. Capacity for some dependency relationship.
      i. Capacity for having worked out compensatory drives for inadequacies.

2. Setting for interview.
   a. Appointment.
   b. Time allotted.
   c. Preoccupation at time of interview.
   d. Environment.
   e. Presence of other persons.
3. Personality factors of interviewee and social worker determined by:
   a. Status of language, race, education, age, religious attachments.
   b. Quality of imagination, sense of humor, perception, tact, poise, judgment, insight, capacity to see alternatives, objectivity, ethical viewpoint.
   c. Nature of defenses, reaction to physical handicap, instability, fears, prejudices, false beliefs, etc.
   d. Attitudes as they appear to be manifested by voice, gesture, manner, bearing, expressed ideas.

B. Approach.
1. Relationship between interviewee and worker influenced by worker's role of participation which stimulates interviewee:
   a. To a frank reciprocal discussion.
   b. To an expression of problems and plans.
2. Procedures.
   a. Depending upon interviewee's response and ability to participate:
      1. In worker's control of situation:
         a. Obtain interviewee's statement of his needs and expectations from the agency.
         b. Interpret agency to interviewee.
         c. Explain reason for direct questions or notations.
         d. Consider time element:
            (1) By creating appearance of ease.
            (2) By stating need for time.
            (3) In meeting issues.
         e. Use language within interviewee's educational grasp.
         f. Assume the obvious.

g. Be non-committal to bring out interviewee's reaction.

h. Allow discussion of interviewee's misapprehensions and prejudices without defensive reactions on part of worker.

i. Repeat opportunity for release of interviewee's hostilities.

j. Recognize interviewee's potentialities and limitations and indicate possibilities for achievement.

k. Maintain an understanding attitude while interviewee carries through his plan if practical, giving interviewee opportunity to
  (1) Make plans.
  (2) Make decisions.
  (3) Change mind.
  (4) Present objections.

l. Stimulate by discussion to a new objective when plan presented is not feasible, leaving freedom for initiative to interviewee:
  (1) Allow interviewee's interpretation of the facts to explain motives for his actions.
  (2) Appraise and indicate irrefutable facts as previously given by interviewee to enable him to draw own conclusions.
  (3) Point out other possibilities.

m. Develop self-esteem.
  (1) Avoid painful recollections.
  (2) Review past progress.

n. Encourage mutual understanding.

o. Present a practical goal.

p. Consider giving definite advice and information regarding the meeting of specific needs.

q. Evade issues when advisable.

r. Avoid humiliation, ridicule, nagging, argumentation, threats, use of detective methods and coercion.

s. Use authority only.

(1) When an interviewee is unable to make a necessary decision.
(2) As a protection of interviewee.
(3) As a therapeutic measure.
(4) As a protection of community.

2. In stimulating interest and discussion:

a. Appeal to reason and imagination, the emotions and sentiments, such as humor, pride and approbation, sense of fairness and religious feelings, affection and sympathy, respectability and individual integrity.

b. Show appreciation of interviewee's efforts by:

(1) Agreeing when possible.
(2) Expressing approbation when advisable.
(3) Selecting favorable elements of the situation.

c. Gradual encouragement of interviewee's initiative.

d. Suggestion when advisable.

e. Repetition.

3. In understanding resistance of interviewee by:

a. Universalizing of problem when advisable.
b. Changing of approach.
c. Explaining need of coöperation.
d. Helping him face his lack of coöperation.
e. Supporting interviewee's point of view whenever desirable.

4. In facing and accepting reality:

a. Allow opportunity for interviewee's expression of problem with minimum of stimulation.

b. Assure respect of confidence to stimulate the expression of confidential information.

c. Enable interviewee to see his problem in relation to his other experiences and his meeting of these.

d. Cite comparative illustration from worker's knowledge and experience when advisable.

e. Mutually evaluate and interpret situation according to degree of interviewee's emotional acceptance.

f. Mutually appraise interviewee's personality equipment to enable him to recognize and use constructively.

g. Develop questioning attitude in interviewee's mind with the idea of eventually changing his point of view.

h. Give general information from worker's experience and knowledge to stimulate application to specific problem by interviewee.

i. Reorganize ideas and experiences to affect new behavior.

b. When interviewee is emotionally upset:

1. Recognize interviewee's emotional state with appreciation of its possibilities.

2. Ease situation by tolerant understanding, by not expressing judgment on issues, by analyzing a general statement, by generalizing specific statements.

3. Start discussion of problem with least irritating aspect.

4. Help interviewee regain self-control after a difficult emotional interview.

a. Avoid centering upon emotional reactions.

b. Allow expression of and minimize reasons for fear, shame or stigma when advisable.

c. Ignore emotional reactions of patient accustomed to gaining an end by that method.

3. General attitudes influencing worker's methods:

a. Respect interviewee's integrity.

b. Assume coöperation on part of interviewee.
c. Keep responsiveness and understanding of interviewee's mood.
d. Establish understanding on basis of tolerance and objectivity.
e. Manifest same attitude toward interviewee's problem as would be desirable for interviewee to assume.
f. Accept interviewee's display of emotion with understanding.
g. Admit errors.

C. Analysis of:
1. Delineation of patient's attitude as expressed towards the problem, environment, personality and plans.
2. Social worker's interpretation of interviewee's attitude and her own in the meeting of those by:
   a. Anticipation of her rôle in relationship with interviewee.
   b. Awareness of problem and question of revealing her knowledge of such to interviewee.
   c. Ability to gauge the time of interviewee's receptivity.
3. Social worker's plans by
   a. Constant evaluation of procedure and progess by
      1. Worker.
      2. Group discussion.
   b. Directed experimentation.

D. Treatment.
1. Aims.
   a. Immediate.
      1. Establishing for interviewee:
         a. A contact with worker which gives him security.
         b. A realization, at least in part, of his contribution to problem.
         c. A willingness to coöperate in treatment of problem.
      2. Establishing for worker's clarification:
         a. Early analysis of material available to

formulate social diagnosis and prognosis.

b. A concept of emotional and social factors and attitudes involved in the problem.

c. Early defining of objectives relative to individual needs of case and consideration of focus of treatment.

b. Ultimate.

1. Developing interviewee's understanding of causes for problem.

2. Developing interviewee's ability to plan in view of his insight gained.

3. Interviewee's ability to modify attitude and conduct in view of insight gained.

2. Types.

a. Symptomatic—A teaching relationship, the use of which is based on determining factors such as:

1. Type of individual interviewed—a person temporarily or permanently incapable of developing or using insight in working out his problem.

a. Emotionally upset.

b. Psychotic.

c. Mentally defective.

d. Delinquent.

e. Chronically unstable.

2. Type and limitations of agency.

a. Time.

b. Case-load pressure.

c. Personnel.

3. As a planned approach to more intensive treatment:

a. To relieve acute problem first.

b. To develop understanding and discussion on part of interviewee.

b. Dynamic—A therapeutic relationship based on determining factors such as:

1. Potentialities of interviewee:

a. His recognition of a problem and of his responsibility for the problem.

b. His willing acceptance of treatment offered by worker.

c. His ability to relate and associate past experiences with present problems and to develop objectivity for use of insight gained.

2. Potentialities of worker based on:

a. Training.

b. Experience.

c. Personality.

d. Ability to guide and evaluate interviewee's expression and understanding of interrelationships in problems, as far as his acceptance is possible.

E. Evaluation of social treatment—To be used in analyzing changes of attitude that have occurred where treatment was focussed:

1. On whom was treatment focussed and reasons for choice.
2. Compare interviewee's concept of the problem at admission to present concept of problem.
3. What were interviewee's first expectations from treatment.
4. What and how much does interviewee recognize as his contribution to the problem.
5. What responsibility has interviewee taken for treatment of the problem.
6. What use did interviewee make of treatment relationships:

a. Did he seek suggestion, advice, information, specific service, authority.

b. Did he escape responsibility by means of:

1. Dependency on worker.

2. Evasion of problem.

c. Did he use relationship as a means to gain his ends destructively.

d. Did he gain emotional release by expressing feelings and attitudes, regarding problem, regarding himself.

e. Did he seek specific or general interpretation.

   f. Did he seek mutual study and understanding of the problem.
   g. Did he seek treatment of self.
7. Evaluate from record the nature of worker's approach with interviewee; whether, when and extent used:
   a. Educational or teaching—interpretation, suggestion or advice.
   b. Therapeutic—a medium to provide:
      1. Release of emotion.
      2. Discussion largely directed by interviewee with leads from worker by which conclusions and mutual interpretations were drawn.
   c. Methods used by worker to control interview and reasons for selection.
8. Interviewee's contribution to treatment:
   a. Ability to discuss spontaneously:
      1. By complaints.
      2. By relating history.
      3. By relating recent episodes and problems.
      4. By discourse on self.
   b. Ability in light of his experience to discover and relate cause and effect; e.g., emotional factors producing problem.
   c. Ability to recognize emotional needs of those concerned in problem.
   d. Interviewee's resourcefulness in planning.
   e. Interviewee's ability to develop objectivity.
   f. Practicability of interviewee's plans in view of insight gained; e.g., satisfaction of emotional needs of those involved.
9. Consideration of extraneous factors contributing to or limiting treatment:
   a. Within worker's control.
   b. Within interviewee's control.
   c. Outside worker's or interviewee's control.
10. Direct or indirect treatment among family members other than person on whom treatment is focussed and effects gained.
11. Evaluation of treatment results:

a. Quantitative—What immediate and ultimate aims of treatment were accomplished.
b. Qualitative—Factors influencing treatment results:
   1. Worker's comparative understanding of problem:
      a. Initial concept.
      b. Present concept.
   2. Worker's adaptations of treatment to problem.
   3. Amount of correlation in treatment process between psychiatrist and worker and corresponding effects upon those treated.
      a. Consider progress in treatment affecting patient and affecting interviewee upon whom social treatment is focussed.
         (1) Relationship of patient's treatment, if any, upon response and treatment with interviewee.
         (2) Interviewee's changed expectations of treatment, if any, in view of treatment progress.
      b. Interviewee's acceptance and understanding of patient's recovery or present problem, if any, in view of treatment progress.
   4. Amount of correlation in treatment process between psychiatrist and worker if both are treating patient.
      a. Type of service rendered by each.
      b. Results obtained.
   5. Worker's estimate of outstanding personality traits in interviewee, limiting or contributing to treatment. (pp. 7-17)

There are certain factors in the hospital that have a pronounced influence on the quality of social work, and the type of organization is one of the most important. In the atmosphere of an autocratic form of government, with a dictator-superintendent who seeks to regulate the intellectual thought of the professional group, we invariably find the history-taking, fact-finding, errand-girl kind of social worker. Case work is handicapped by administrative prejudices, legal technicalities, and cautious conservatism. The supervision of the discharged patient is apt to consist of perfunctory family visiting, with little understanding on the part of the worker of what the psychiatrist hopes to accomplish. She rarely knows what her place is in the work of treating the patient and family. On the investigative side she is a psychiatric Sherlock Holmes, looking for clues which show abnormal behavior to confirm a diagnosis. Frequently the psychiatrist pays little attention to her findings because the diagnosis has been made and he has become interested in another "acute case." The acquisition of facts in the patient's history is an important procedure, but unless these facts are utilized to aid the patient directly, the time and energy expended in getting them is wasted. Social service should be an important part of the training of every new staff member. This should not be confined to a course of lectures on theory but should include actual case work under the supervision of a well-trained worker. It is only by actual experience of this kind that the young psychiatrist will acquire the social sense which enables him to utilize the assistance of the worker in the study and treatment of his cases.

A factor in the failure of psychiatrist and social worker to work in harmony is a lack of understanding of each other's problems. The social worker does not have the knowledge of hospital ideals and routine that enables her to interpret properly the organization to the community. This is the fault of the administrator. She should be properly instructed in these matters. Questions of principles and policy should be given to her by the superintendent and the therapeutic routine should be explained to her by the ward psychiatrist. Psychiatrists may be uncoöperative with social workers because of their own emotional insecurity. They feel that it is an admission of inferiority to permit anyone to know more about the patient than they do. Medical men have fostered a tradition that no one should be permitted to do anything for the sick individual except the physician, and the psychiatrist who is not secure in his belief of the efficacy of his own ministrations may see the social worker as a menace to this well-established tradition.

There is the psychiatrist who interprets the work of the social worker as a function entirely separate from his responsibility. Having referred the patient to her, he gives no further thought to the matter. It becomes her problem. This "buck-passing" attitude is a danger that is always present, and frequently the coördinating guidance of the superintendent is needed to get real harmony into the relationship. The social worker makes her best contribution where she has the complete sympathy and understanding of the professional staff. Without this her position is intolerable and the well-trained, self-respecting worker will not struggle against such odds. The social worker does not work for the psychiatrist. She works with him and both work for the patient.

If the patient is to receive the benefit that comes from social treatment, it can only be made available through a partnership arrangement of psychiatrist and social worker. Such a union will lead to the development of a therapeutic program for both patient and family that will carry on throughout the hospital residence. The psychiatrist and worker, having a mutual respect and a complete understanding of each other's profession, will pool their knowledge for the good of the patient. Such relationship ideally develops best in a democratic type or organization where the standards of psychiatry are high and where the organization is built around the idea of therapy.

DEPARTMENTAL ORGANIZATION

Qualifications of Social Workers. It is exceedingly difficult to outline the qualifications of age, education, and training for professional people who deal with human material, but a lack of definite standards for hospital social workers is one of the reasons for the inability of the psychiatrist to see the worker in her proper position. Mediocre and poorly trained individuals do not interpret the ideals of the social work to psychiatrists as they should. Workers of inferior educational background are not acceptable as equals, and where equality does not exist there can be little real coöperation. Naturally the qualifications demanded by the administrator will depend largely upon his idea of social work. If he has the older conception, the qualifications need only be those possessed by any experienced social worker or even a well-trained public health nurse. Either of these can acquire the familiarity with hospital organization, the knowledge of mental symptoms, and the necessary fluency of psychiatric terminology which will enable her to carry on within narrow limits. If, however, the administrator desires an individual who can deal with the personality of the patient in his social situation, who can interpret correctly mental mechanisms to the family, and who has the ability to be a real member of the psychiatric team, he will require a very different general and professional background.

The educational qualifications as outlined by the American Association of Psychiatric Social Workers are as follows:

An A.B. degree or its equivalent is required for membership. Graduates of recognized courses in psychiatric social work of not less than nine months' duration are eligible after they have held a position in psychiatric social work for one year; graduates of other recognized training courses in social work of not less than nine months' duration are eligible after they have held a position in psychiatric social work for at least two years; and persons who have not taken formal training but have met certain educational requirements and substitutes for training are eligible after four years of successful accomplishment in psychiatric social work, if they have entered the field of psychiatric social work prior to January, 1929. These are the membership requirements of the psychiatric social workers' professional organization.

In the selection of social workers the administrator will do well to follow these requirements closely. For head workers who have charge of the department, additional qualifications and training along organization lines will be essential. She will be responsible for the quality of case work carried on, the training of personnel, and the general administration of the department. The work carried on will be no better or no worse than she will permit. Upon her ability and experience rests the social service program of the hospital. As to her general personality traits, it is more difficult to make dogmatic statements. One who is emotionally unstable and immature starts with a great handicap when she attempts to unravel the tangled threads in the life of someone else.

In this connection I quote from an article by Dr. Jessie Taft[27] on the "Qualifications of The Social Worker":

"The born social worker has to be a maternal sort of person even if she is only twenty. She has to have a genuine liking for people and their troubles. She needs a warmth and spontaneity and whole-hearted interest that render the making of good contacts simple, natural, and inevitable. She should be a settled person, fairly satisfied, who has a philosophy of life which she has tried out and can pass on with conviction and whose basic attitude towards life is a sober optimism. Without this she will not find it easy to throw her interest into the problems of every patient with perfect objectivity. The restless, unfulfilled, seeking, pessimistic individual cannot tear her attention loose from her own troubles long enough to manage other people's. And finally, the ideal psychiatric social worker must be the person who has strength to carry the patient, the poise which gives him confidence, the sympathy that means real understanding, the open mind which is always ready to try a new plan, the wisdom to allow the patient to work out his own salvation as far as he can, and the unending patience which is the rock on which he depends."

The director must be a recognized member of the hospital professional staff. If her qualifications, training, and experience conform to the accepted standard and her personality enables her to work comfortably in a coöperative enterprise, she will be accepted by the group. But if she is an individual of mediocre training and background or if she has a difficult personality, all the administrative support in the world will not give her the status her position calls for.

Quota of Personnel

Figures regarding the proper ratio of social workers to hospital population are almost entirely lacking. There are so many factors which change with local conditions that it seems impossible to arrive at any satisfactory ratio that will fit all institutions. Distances and transportation facilities must always be taken into consideration in establishing a fair case load.

The thickly settled territory of the eastern seaboard, where the population is urban, creates very different problems from the sparsely settled areas of the middle west, where the communities are rural. Clerical facilities must be thought of. The more active the department the greater the amount of clerical work which is needed. It is not economical to make a social worker spend her time writing records, filing cases, and doing work for which she is not qualified and which can be carried on more efficiently by lower-salaried employees. The type of social work to be done would regulate quotas to a large extent. The administrator whose social service ideals call for intensive therapeutic work with patients and relatives will need more workers than the one who is primarily interested in "after care."

Many other considerations enter into this matter of the number of workers. The subject deserves more study than it has been given. At present any figures stated are based purely on individual experience and impressions. It is the belief of the writer that the number of workers should be based on admission rate rather than hospital population. The best information available would indicate that for intensive psychiatric social work, a case load of 50 patients per worker is sufficient where distances are not too great. But it can be safely assumed that a certain number of patients admitted will not need such intensive work, and this can be set at one-half of the admissions. Therefore, a figure of one social worker to every 100 admissions would seem to be fairly accurate. It would mean that the hospital with an admission rate of 500 patients annually would have five workers. In the matter of family care, one worker can give proper supervision to 75 patients. Quotas can be based upon the number of patients on visit or parole. Here the ratio should be 1 to 50. Most of these patients require very close and intensive work, and a case load of this size would give each worker a fair amount of work. It should be borne in mind that every worker added increases the cost of travel, clerical help, telephone, and postage. But in my opinion it is worth the additional cost because it will save the per capita expenditure for the maintenance of the patient in the hospital and, what is more important, will lessen the necessity for additional construction. If one worker can keep 50 patients out of the hospital, why should we quibble over an additional number. There is no limit until we meet the law of diminishing returns, and I see no danger of the operation of the law yet.

SOCIAL SERVICE A DIVISION OF THE PSYCHIATRIC DEPARTMENT

Social service must be an integral part of the psychiatric work of the hosptial if it is to achieve the maximum amount of good for the patient. It cannot be an isolated unit. In order to secure the effect of bringing worker and psychiatrist closer together, some consideration must be given to the physical conditions under which they work. To discuss this it is necessary to go into the matter of medical staff organization.

In my experience the central office used by the medical staff in many of the older institutions does not serve the best interests of the hospital. The closer the psychiatrist is to his patients, the more they occupy his thought and attention. The better he can supervise and direct the work of his assistants, the more efficient his organization is. If we concede that therapeutic efforts are improved through the establishment of a psychiatric team under the guidance and leadership of the psychiatrist, we must believe that all members of this team should have the closest relationship with him. The more difficult of access he is, the less rapport there is between himself and the group. For this reason it seems that a decentralization of the psychiatric and allied departments is the desirable arrangement. And here I can only state the principle and not the method. Such organization depends so much upon the physical lay-out of the hospital and the possibilities of finding available office space that it would be impertinent for anyone to suggest details. What would be efficient in one institution would be entirely impractical in another. But the principle of eliminating the old-time central medical office and substituting offices for psychiatrists nearer the wards they serve is, in my opinion, a progressive change. Every mental hospital is divided into male and female services. Usually each service is in charge of a senior physician. In the newer hospitals the admission service is a separate unit, but divided into sexes as is the rest of the institution. Each of these services should be a completely organized unit under the control of the psychiatrist. His office should be in the center of this group and all should be easily accessible to each other. Who are the members of the psychiatric team? First, of course, comes the psychiatrist who is in charge of the service. He is the leader and coördinator and is the one who is responsible to the clinical director and through him to the superintendent and medical council. All of his psychiatric assistants, junior staff members, internes, and students, are a part of the team. The representative of the nursing group in charge of the service is an important member. This would be the chief supervisor, and her office should be in close proximity to that of the psychiatrist. The social service office should be adjacent to the medical section. Other members of this psychiatric team are the occupational therapist and the psychologist who is assigned to the service. The latter has no office but attends all conferences and has the work of the service as her major responsibility. We have, then, a group under the direction and leadership of the psychiatrist, working in close contact with each other and available for frequent conference. It is a psychiatric unit responsible for the complete therapy of the service. As many units can be organized as there are services. Some administrators may object to this method of organization on the basis that it has a divided responsibility. The social worker is under the control of the psychiatrist while at the same time she has a direct contact with the director of social service. The latter supervises the quality of case work and student teaching. This type of organization is frequently used in industrial plants. It is known as functional management. Instead of one foreman the workmen may have several, each one responsible for a certain function. A gang boss has charge of the preparation of the work up to the time it is put into the machine, the speed boss is responsible for the correct machining of the work and the time in which it is completed. He is the teacher. An inspector is responsible for the quality of the work and the repair boss is responsible for the maintenance of the machines and for seeing that the workmen keep them in first-class condition. Translated into terms of hospital organization, we have all professional workers under the direct supervision of the psychiatrist. He decides what cases are most important, what the psychiatric implications are, and what part

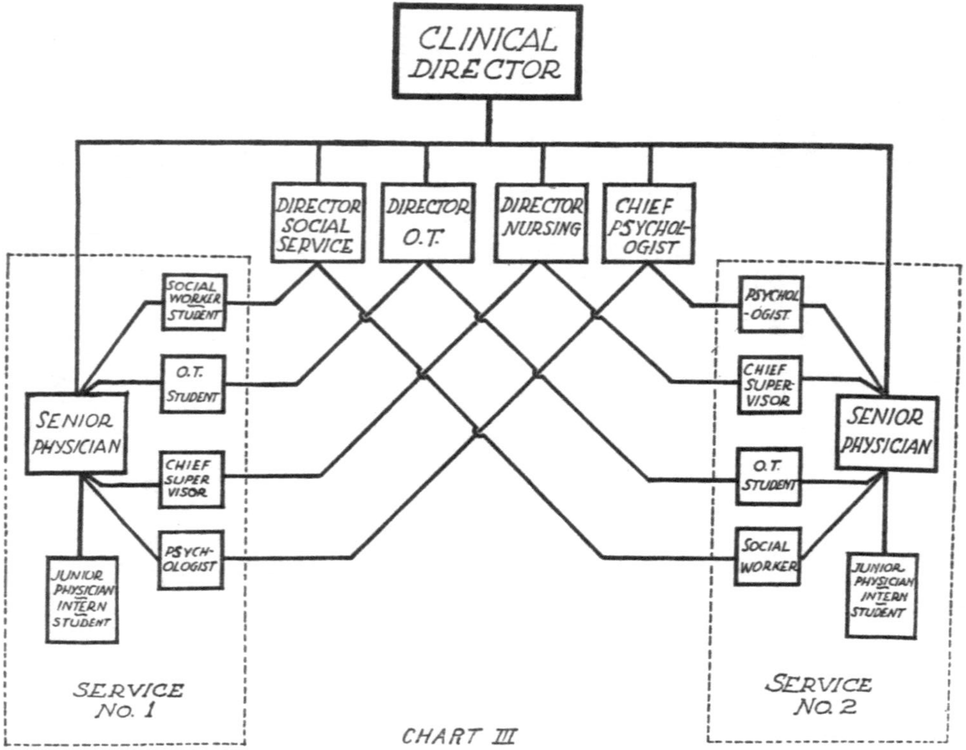
CLINICAL DIRECTOR
DIRECTOR SOCIAL SERVICE
DIRECTOR O.T.
DIRECTOR NURSING
CHIEF PSYCHOL-OGIST
SOCIAL WORKER STUDENT
O.T. STUDENT
SENIOR PHYSICIAN
CHIEF SUPER VISOR
PSYCH-OLOGIST
JUNIOR PHYSICIAN INTERN STUDENT
SERVICE No. 1
PSYCHOL-OGIST
CHIEF SUPER-VISOR
SENIOR PHYSICIAN
O.T. STUDENT
SOCIAL WORKER
JUNIOR PHYSICIAN INTERN STUDENT
SERVICE No. 2

CHART III

of the treatment each should undertake. The director of social service is held responsible for the quality of the case work done, the kind of teaching that students receive, and their assignment to special cases. She is the teacher rather than the administrator.

This type of organization tends to break down the barrier that exists between psychiatrist and social worker when everything has to pass through the director's hands. Red tape must be eliminated if there is to be real coöperation. The psychiatrist must be easily available to all social workers in his unit for conferences on cases. He must recognize his responsibility to them in the matter of psychiatric guidance and be resourceful and ingenious in pointing out new ways of approach and different methods of handling difficult situations. The unit should have a daily staff meeting on cases on which work is being done. These unit conferences may well take the place of the usual mental hospital staff meetings where much time is spent quibbling over diagnostic abstractions. All unit staff meetings deal largely with progress of therapy. The entire program for the treatment of the patient should be the product of the unit.

The following therapeutic program is a sample of the kind of record produced under the unit form of administration:

PRESENT AT CONFERENCE:

Senior Psychiatrist
Internist
Social Worker
Occupational Therapist
Supervisor of Nursing
Psychologist

The diagnosis made is general paresis. Prognosis favorable.

OUTLINE OF THERAPY

1. Patient to be placed on diathermy treatment at once. To remain on the medical service until the series is completed, which will be within two weeks.

2. Social service to contact family for two purposes:

   A. To bring the wife to the point where she will permit an examination of her blood and that of the children.

B. To change her attitude about the patient's illness. She is very bitter towards him and needs much re-education.

3. The psychiatrist to see the patient at least three times a week. He is depressed because of his disease and on account of his wife's attitude towards him. Such superficial psychotherapy will help correct his depression.

4. The internist to enlist the aid of the physiotherapy technician to encourage the patient and try to change his attitude towards the situation.

5. The occupational therapist to start the patient in the pre-industrial class two hours each day to get him ready to be placed in the mattress shop.

All of these procedures were based upon an accurate social history of the case. The patient is not only suffering from an actual pathological condition but the entire family is in a social situation that needs careful treatment. Of what avail will it be to correct the physical difficulty and leave the social damage? We must make an effort to patch up the wreck.

RECORDS

The case record of every patient should contain all the material on that patient. This means that all social service findings, correspondence, and medical examinations are filed as part of the psychiatric record, which is available for every member of the unit. Through this medium the psychiatrist cannot overlook the social service report and the social worker will know more about the psychiatric mechanisms that are involved. When social service records are buried in special files they are not utilized to the fullest extent. Everything should be arranged to merge the psychiatric and social interests. Such records will contain the nursing observations, psychological reports, and occupational therapy progress notes. It should have a complete account of all therapy so that every member of the unit may know what other therapies are being carried on.

STANDARD PRACTICE

The following standard practice shows the close affiliation of the social service division with the other professional departments of the hospital.

MEDICAL STAFF

Superintendent. Function—executive. To be consulted only on major matters, particularly on questions of hospital policy or on unusually serious problems that are of concern to the worker or the hospital.

Assistant Superintendent. Function—administrative. To be consulted on difficult cases where community relationship is involved and on problems which relate to other departments of the hospital.

Clinical Director. Function—educational. To be consulted in special cases, particularly with regard to those involving medical, psychiatric, or neurological problems of which the worker has little knowledge.

Director of Clinics. Function—supervisor of all out-patient work. To be consulted in cases where the behavior of children and adults in the community is in question.

Physicians. To be consulted before visiting patients on the wards. Each case to be discussed with the physician before the medical-social history is taken, in order to determine what points are to be emphasized in getting the history. Plans for the patient who is to be released are to be discussed with the physician and he is to be kept in touch with the progress of the patient outside the hospital. Workers should refer all inquiries regarding the physical or mental condition of the patient to the psychiatrist.

NURSING STAFF

Director of Nursing. To be consulted regarding contacts with nurses.

Nurses. To be consulted regarding their observations of patients, both as to information for medical-social histories and condition of patients for discharge.

CLERICAL STAFF

Head Clerk. Function—in charge of files and records of patients. To be consulted regarding commitment matters. Stenographers are procured through her.

FINANCIAL DEPARTMENT

Treasurer. To be consulted about all money matters of patients. No money should be collected or accepted for patients without first consulting her. Monthly expenses must be in the office of the Treasurer, signed and receipted, before noon of the last day of the month.

Vouchers—must be handed in with monthly report of travel and hotel bills, as well as money spent for car expenses.

Matron. To be consulted regarding room and personal comfort.

OFFICE ROUTINE

Time Schedule. Each worker is to have a regular hour for consultation with the head worker. Her time for visits and office work is to be planned according to schedule, as far as possible. She will have responsibility for the office on regularly assigned days.

Day Sheet. Records of visits are to be entered daily on the day sheet. These are used to make up the monthly report.

Notices. Are to be signed after worker has read them and passed on.

Bulletin Board. To be consulted daily for current notices.

Records. No records are to be given out to any individual or agency outside the social service staff.

A. When a social service record is completed it is to be placed on the head worker's desk.

B. Medical-social histories must be completed and in the hands of the head worker by the twelfth day after admission.

C. Notes on visit cases must be written by the 30th of each month.

D. No records are to be left in the social service office after 5:00 P.M. When records are required after this hour they may be obtained at the telephone office.

E. Requests for discharged cases must be approved by the head worker.

FAMILY CARE

The idea of community care for mental patients has been in existence for many years, both in this country and in Europe. The famous Gheel Colony is the most conspicuous example of family care of the insane. It is likewise the oldest system in the world. Scotland, France, and Sweden have had "boarding out" for many years. In Colonial New England, before state hospitals were in existence, towns contracted with families to care for the "pauper insane." No standards were set and no supervision was given.

The Scotch plan of boarding mental patients in the community came out of the work of Dorothea Dix. As a result of her visit to Scotland in 1857, a board of commissioners in lunacy was organized. The first work of the board was to make a survey to determine what provision should be made for mental patients. The decision was that many patients should be cared for without being committed, while others, after a brief sojourn in the institution, could be returned to private homes. During the years 1885-89, as many as 60 per cent of the patients under care were boarded with private families. The 1930 annual report of the General Board of Control for Scotland shows that 1,124, or 34 per cent, of the total number of insane were cared for in private homes. The Scotch system offered certain advantages over other plans. The question of supervision was carefully worked out. Patients are visited once each year by the assistant commissioner, who is an ex-superintendent of a mental hospital, twice each year by the overseer of the poor, and every three months by a physician who is appointed for the purpose.

There was much opposition in this country to the use of private homes for mental patients. Many questions were raised and the same doubts are expressed today. Most of the opposition came from psychiatric administrators. Some felt that the patients would have a deleterious effect upon the family, that the individual members would take on the peculiarities of the patients. The danger of neglect on the part of the caretakers was pointed out. It was argued that while the Scotch peasant might be willing to keep patients for a mere pittance, American farmers would not be so ready to act as guardians for mental patients. A few believed that too much supervision would be required of the caretakers. One superintendent objected to the plan on the grounds that it would take too much labor away from the institutions and another sarcastically recommended that the advocates of the plan learn more about the insane. All of these questions are raised today.

In the *American Journal of Insanity*, April, 1869,[28] the Scotch system is discussed, the purposes of the plan being listed as follows:

A. Placing the mental patient in sane society.
B. Training him to some industrial pursuit.
C. Allowing him more personal liberty and nearer approximation to the ordinary mode of social life.

The following shows the type of patients that were selected: "Those patients whose mental impairment consists of the milder forms of melancholia, of moral or emotional insanity, which while they deprive them of the faculty of entire self-government and unfit them for responsibilities and more or less for the pursuits of life, neither destroy the reasoning powers, deaden the sensibilities nor introduce any element of danger into the outer or inner life. Those chronic cases in which some harmless, fixed delusion, the residuum of a more pervading active form of insanity, co-exists with much power of general self-regulation and an intelligent appreciation of the concern and interests of normal life. Those patients who are liable to occasional or periodical attacks of acute disorder but who have long intervals of partial sanity."

This general classification can be used today in the selection of patients who are suitable for family care.

After many years of discussion an act was passed by the Massachusetts legislature which provided for the boarding out of mental patients in private families. Massachusetts followed the Scotch plan with some modifications. For example, no patient is placed in a boarding home without first having been committed to a mental hospital. In this way it is possible to gain some understanding of the patient and his needs before he is placed in family care. Patients are not boarded with their relatives at the expense of the state.

For many years the boarding home has been used largely for the care of a custodial type of patient, but more recently the system has developed along different lines. Family care is now being tried as a therapeutic measure, and it is the personal opinion of the writer that the system will become a very valuable tool for social case work. The use of a boarding home has proven very successful as an aid in the readjustment of certain psychotic patients in the community.

The selection of the home, or rather the caretaker, is the first consideration. The human elements in the home are of vastly greater importance than the physical set-up. Adequate physical care is essential, including good food and a comfortable room which may or may not be shared by another patient but not with a member of the family. But if these boarding homes are to have a therapeutic value, the personality of the caretaker and each member of the family is of greatest importance. Every member of the family group has an influence on the patient. Each one must be studied and understood by the social worker and reckoned as an asset or liability in the treatment of the patient. The general spirit of the home and the amount of harmony and coöperation are far more important than modern conveniences.

The caretaker who is overburdened with personal problems is not a good caretaker. She has insufficient time and energy to give to the problems of the patients. Financial difficulties do not necessarily disqualify, but worry, fear of losing the home, and financial insecurity great enough to absorb the family interest react unfavorably on the patient, not necessarily because they exploit him but because he shares the sorrows and worries as well as the joys of the group in which he is living.

A second important factor in the family care system is the selection of the patient for a particular home. Family care offers the convalescent psychotic an opportunity to become accustomed to community life without the entanglements of personal and family problems, such as would be present in his own home. But it is important that neither family nor patient should be permitted to feel that the boarding home is the final solution to his problems. The pressure to become again a self-sustaining member of society must always be on him. While boarding out will always be used for certain chronic patients who require kindly and humane custodial care, the main emphasis in the future should be therapy. Such ideals require careful supervision and intensive case work which will lead to financial and emotional independence. And while this kind of supervision may be more expensive for a time, in the end it is economical because it leads to recovery.

In general we find that the schizophrenic makes the best adjustment in a simple situation. Depressed patients are more unhappy in a home where there is confusion and excitement. But other patients may thrive in such an atmosphere.

Experience has demonstrated that patients can adjust to a lower level than that to which they have been accustomed. But attempts to place them in homes that are better than their own have invariably ended in failure. It is not good policy to attempt to raise the standards too much. Frequently homes that consider other matters of more value than having perfect order are highly beneficial for certain patients. But those who are orderly in their habits become very unhappy when placed in homes that are indifferent in this respect.

Every attempt should be made to bring the caretaker to the realization that she is a part of the hospital organization.

This may be accomplished to some extent by bringing all caretakers to the institution several times a year for instruction by the psychiatrist. A program is arranged, followed by a discussion period. Problems dealing with particular patients may be discussed. In our experience it has been found desirable to select several homes in the same community. It is in this way that community spirit is built up and the work becomes a part of the group interest. The patient ceases to be an object of curiosity but is accepted by others on a more normal level.

There are many arguments offered against this tool for social case work. The success or failure of boarding out depends, in a large measure, upon the degree of intelligent supervision which the patients receive. From the humanitarian point of view, no one could visit a group of patients in a boarding home and ever feel that they would be better off in the bustle and confusion of a mental hospital. The normal level of life on which they live, the quiet, peaceful surroundings of a good home, and the tranquillizing effect of community life does bring peace and happiness into the lives of certain mental patients even though they do not entirely recover from their psychosis. Even if the per capita cost were higher than hospital care it would still be economical because it decreases the need for additional construction. It offers an excellent way by which states can relieve, to some extent, the overcrowding.

Social service has become an indispensable part of the therapeutic program of the modern, progressive mental hospital. The worker is an important member of the psychiatric team and administrators may well emphasize the need of well-trained and qualified professional workers in every mental hospital. If one social worker can keep fifty patients out of the hospital there should be no limit to the number employed except a saturation point. But until the law of diminishing returns operates, I advocate the employment of more and more workers.

Chapter 10

THE TEACHING PROGRAM

WHY should the mental hospital carry on a teaching program?

How may it be done efficiently and not interfere with patient care and treatment?

Whom shall we teach?

What should be taught?

These are some of the questions which will arise in the minds of many administrators who give thought to this problem. There are those who say that the primary purpose of the hospital is to care for sick people, that the responsibility for teaching belongs to the educational institution and each should look after its own business. With this point of view no one can quarrel. But applied literally, it becomes narrow and short-sighted. Others maintain that the hospital has neither time nor organization to develop an educational scheme. This is true to a considerable extent as the mental institution is set up today. But that it need always be true is a debatable point. It is my thesis that patient care and teaching are not incompatible but, on the contrary, the teaching hospital from a therapeutic viewpoint is superior to the one which does not have an educational outlook. The mere presence of a group of young students—interested, enthusiastic, with high ideals, and intellectually alive—prevents hospital inertia, the bane of every progressive administrator. Teaching and being taught stimulates every member of the professional staff and keeps the entire organization on the *qui vive*. The sum total of the group reaction to an educational program is to place the patient and his needs on a higher plane. With psychiatrically trained ward nurses, the staff physician can multiply himself many times. When he spends a portion of his time teaching, instructing, and guiding these nurses in the field of psychotherapy, he finds that he can accomplish more than would ever be possible working as an individual psychiatrist.

While I do not believe that psychiatry is the answer to all

problems in life, I am convinced that a psychiatric approach to the understanding of human behavior should be utilized more extensively than it is by all workers in the fields of physiological, social, and psychological maladaptation. The emphasis upon the human being as a total organism and the consideration of him as an individual in relation to his physical and social environment should be thoughtfully considered by all disciplines whose representatives attempt to deal with people. Psychiatry cannot be learned from books and didactic lectures. It must come as the result of actual contact with patients. Theories may be discussed in the classroom, but when we attempt to fit them to conditions as they are, something is missing. And that something is the skill and understanding which can be acquired only through the medium of clinical experience. Much of our physiological, social, and psychological knowledge has come from the study of the abnormal. Medicine, as a result of the understanding of pathological phenomena, has been able to make great progress in the field of prevention. Social service has learned the causes of maladjustment from those who have failed at the social level. Psychology is indebted to the feebleminded for the development of psychometry. And mental hygiene was born of the recognition that the patient with mental disease is only an exaggeration of his own normal, personal self. Mental mechanisms cannot be studied with any degree of success in healthy people. The inhibitions which prevent one from getting a glimpse of the individual's inner mental and emotional life create difficulties that cannot be overcome. In the psychotic these restraints have, in large part, disappeared and the student can study the emotional and intellectual processes in "pure culture." Therefore the State hospital is in the unique position of having under strict control conditions great groups of psychotic patients who comprise a vast laboratory for the better understanding of human behavior. It is the only place where such excellent facilities are available.

There is a real need for the development of educational centers where psychiatry in its application to the problems of life can be taught through clinical experience. The demand for this service comes from many quarters—medicine, nursing, social service, theology, psychology, sociology. The social sciences are interested in the field because they believe it has something definite to offer. They are anxious to have students get a first-hand knowledge of the techniques with the eventual goal of adapting them to the social problems with which they deal. If the mental hospitals will prepare to meet this need, they will be in a position to make a substantial contribution to social and health education.

The state-controlled psychiatric institutions of this country have approximately 350,000 patients under treatment, many of whom remain for a long period of time. This enables the student to study the variations of conduct and observe the different phases of a psychosis as they are demonstrated in the same individual. The motivating force behind the unusual act is the essence of the matter, and it is essential that the student be in sufficiently good rapport over a long time to dig down below the presenting symptoms and look at the personality upon which they have developed. It is only by doing this that he can apply his psychiatric knowledge to the difficulties of those with whom he deals in his professional work. The psychopathic hospital or the psychiatric department of the general hospital do not have this particular advantage. Because of the high admission rate and small bed capacity, they have become diagnostic clearing points. The student cannot carry out a prolonged study, nor can he follow through a therapeutic program.

The physical plant, equipment, and organization of the State hospitals represent a tremendous financial investment and it is uneconomical not to make use of them to the fullest extent. A teaching relationship between hospital and school would not only save money but would be a powerful factor in the field of prevention. Such a coöperative enterprise would be a valuable contribution to public health. Progress will be accelerated if we bring physicians, nurses, social workers, clergymen, and others into the institution for a sufficient time for them to acquire a grasp on psychiatric problems. They will be able to promote, with understanding, a sane attitude towards mental health in their respective spheres.

Before a successful teaching program can be incorporated

into the hospital organization structure, certain attitudes must be created by the administrator in his staff. A recognition that further progress will come only with the assumption of great community responsibility on the part of the institution, a broader outlook, a more optimistic spirit, and the conviction that better service cannot be given by merely building bigger hospitals are all essential to the success of a teaching plan. They must see in student training an opportunity to participate in a mental hygiene program rather than an opportunity to get additional people to do the work without cost. Traditional administration is upset by students. They create new and unusual problems, and the fact that they contribute something vital to the organization is frequently lost sight of.

The administrator must not lose sight of the fact that all disciplines have possible contributions to offer in psychiatry. He must welcome the representatives of all social sciences and invite them to use the facilities of the institution. No teaching plan should be built around any one approach. It must be broad, tolerant, and with a respect for all new, sound thought.

The how of such a program offers many difficulties in our present situation. I am familiar with the fact that many mental hospitals are disgracefully undermanned and that they have scarcely enough professional workers to give more than cursory attention to the patients, to say nothing of carrying a teaching burden. With a ratio of 1 physician to 277.9 patients, which is the average in the State hospitals of the United States, there is little time for instruction of students. Therefore, before these demands can be met adequately, administrators will have to change the thinking of control bodies. They will have to work on the theory that more and better-trained professional personnel is the crying need of the mental hospitals. I have dealt with State legislatures too long not to know the heartbreaking task that confronts the executive who seeks to have a program of increased personnel adopted. But I also know that it can be accomplished by a constant emphasis upon the need. As an intelligent legislator once reminded me, "We have been guided in our thinking by your advice and leadership." The policy of increasing bed capacity rather than personnel has been stressed by hospital administrators. Perhaps we have been trying to cure psychotics and cut down the incidence of mental disease by the use of bricks and mortar.

It is essential that a systematic teaching plan be under the control of one individual, whose main business and responsibility it is. Without such centralization we get wasted effort and duplication. Every mental hospital should have a clinical director whose responsibility is twofold:

1. The maintenance of a high standard of psychiatric performance.

2. The creation and coördination of as extensive a teaching program as the resources of the hospital will permit.

The selection of this individual is a matter of great importance and his qualifications should be carefully considered by the administrator. It is essential that he have a broad viewpoint towards the problems of psychiatry and an understanding of all sound methods of approach to the psychoses. He must possess a personality which inspires enthusiasm for therapy and teaching in the staff members. He will be the psychiatric and educational leader of the group. It is he who directs and coördinates the educational policies of the institution.

Teaching is not entirely an affair of the classroom. In fact psychiatry is best taught by actual contact with case material. The clinical director who thoroughly understands pedagogy will stress the importance of carefully supervised case studies. He will devote much time to bedside instruction. Seminar discussion groups, staff meetings, and ward walks are the important means by which students are instructed, and the formal lectures will be a relatively minor factor in the scheme.

The point I wish to stress is that there must be organization and a delegation of responsibility to one individual if the hospital is to teach students. It is not sufficient to invite interested people to live at the institution and browse about at will. The instruction of personnel should be upon a formal basis.

The question of who is to benefit by this psychiatric instruction is an important one. There are many groups, both in the hospital and outside, who would profit by such an experience. Two responsibilities confront the administrator: first, the instruction of hospital personnel; and second, the instruction of students who come from schools for practical experience in psychiatry. If the resources of the institution do not permit both groups, then the superintendent will wisely confine his efforts to his own people.

The following classification of students illustrates the great potentialities for teaching possessed by mental hospitals:

CLASSIFICATION OF STUDENTS

- A. *Hospital Personnel*
  - 1. *Professional Staff*
  - 2. *Ward Personnel*
    - a. Supervisors
    - b. Nurses
    - c. Attendants
    - d. Miscellaneous Ward Workers
  - 3. *Lay Employees*
    - a. Mechanics
    - b. Domestic Workers
    - c. Kitchen and Dining Room Workers
    - d. Farm Employees
- B. *Students from Outside Hospital*
  - 1. *Medical*
    - a. Undergraduates
    - b. Graduate Internes
      - *1.* Medical
      - *2.* Psychiatric
      - *3.* Laboratory
    - c. Technicians
      - *1.* Laboratory
      - *2.* Physiotherapy
      - *3.* X-ray
    - d. Occupational Therapists
  - 2. *Psychology*
    - a. Workers on Special Projects
    - b. Psychological Internes
  - 3. *Social Service*
    - a. Students from Schools
    - b. Volunteer Workers
  - 4. *Social Sciences*
    - a. Theology
    - b. Sociology
  - 5. *Miscellaneous*
    - a. Biometricians
    - b. Dieticians
    - c. Agricultural Students
    - d. All Others.

Hospital Personnel

There can be no valid excuse for the failure of a mental hospital to instruct its own people. Industrial management has learned that the average worker is only about 35 per cent efficient without training. Proper instruction enables him to increase production and earn a higher wage. It has also been pointed out that the employees will, while in the student period, develop a spirit of loyalty and interest in the organization that can be created in no other way.

Again we may profitably adopt an industrial plan. The hospital would gain much in morale and *esprit de corps* if a carefully planned and supervised training course were given to every new worker, regardless of the department for which he or she had been hired. Usually the employee on entering the service is given a book of rules and a personal interview by the head of his department and then assigned directly to the job. He proceeds to get further understanding of his work where and from whom he can, and it is not always the best kind of information. If time allowed, it would be worth while for the institution to require that every employee spend two weeks on the wards, regardless of what his position is. This would give everyone in the organization a better conception of the purpose of the hospital.

The new employee should be subjected to a carefully organized regime. Every attempt should be made to have him come into a friendly and understanding atmosphere. The introduction to his place in the organization is a most critical procedure. This initiation may result in making a valuable addition to the group or it may create a dissatisfied and disgruntled individual. The following plan is offered for the early training of new employees during the two weeks of their ward service:

Orientation Course

1. *Greeting by Superintendent.* Employees frequently work for long periods without knowing the head of the hospital. In his talk he should outline the principles and policies for which the institution stands.

2. *Instruction in Hospital Routine.* A discussion of rules and standard practice. Every institution should have a standard practice manual for the information of both old and new employees.

3. *Inspection Tour Through Hospital.* A trip through the hospital under the guidance of one who is qualified to explain the relationship of the departments gives an understanding of the institution as an organization.

4. *Moving Picture Film Showing Hospital Activities.* Every hospital should have such a film for educational purposes.

5. *History of Psychiatry.* A carefully prepared talk, illustrated by lantern slides, which gives the salient points in the development of psychiatry and psychiatric hospitals.

6. *State and Hospital Organization.* An explanation of the ways by which state governments attempt to meet the problem of mental disease, and particularly the organization of the state in which the hospital is located.

7. *Hospital Organization.* A complete discussion of the hospital organization. A chart is used which shows the lines of responsibilities and promotion.

8. *Hospital Finances.* Includes information regarding the source of the money, methods of appropriating it, budget preparation, waste and control of expenditures. Illustrated by charts and diagrams.

9. *Legal Considerations.* An explanation of the processes of legal commitments, with a discussion of such other laws that may have a bearing on mental disease.

10. *Standards of Patient Care.* A full discussion of those routine matters of custodial care which are the foundation of all methods of treatment.

This course must be presented in simple, non-technical language, and diagrams and charts should be freely used.

NURSE TRAINING

The establishment of nursing schools was a forward step in the field of hospital psychiatry. The movement came at the time when asylums were being converted into hospitals and the influence of the schools was all for the benefit of the patients. The teaching program did much to improve the morale of the hospital organization. Nursing as a profession was in its infancy at the time. But it has now grown into adolescence and while it has the emotional instability of that period, it gives promise of eventually developing into a fine, upstanding citizen and a profession second to none in its health contributions.

The traditional manner of conducting schools of nursing in mental hospitals is to hire students as attendants, place them on wards in positions of responsibility, and give them formal education after their duties as attendants have been fulfilled. There has been no separation of education from ward service. Mental institutions have not taken their educational responsibilities too seriously. They have purported to train nurses for general nursing without the necessary clinical material for proper experience in medicine and surgery, obstetrics and pediatrics. This necessitates an affiliating year in the general hospital. Much of the teaching has been carried on by staff physicians who frequently look upon such duties as an unpleasant chore, to be carried out with the least possible expenditure of time and energy. While occasionally we find a hospital psychiatrist who has the ability and desire to teach nurses, in general the picture is as I have painted it. Pedagogical techniques are not good, there has been little expenditure for equipment, and living quarters for students rarely compare favorably with those of the general hospitals. Such methods have prevented the mental hospital from competing with the well organized general hospital school of nursing, and have tended to bring discredit upon the graduates.

When students are paid salaries as attendants, they are not students but hospital employees. They carry the same responsibility as every other attendant. When they leave the wards for the necessary classroom work, which in many states is extremely heavy, there is a shortage of ward personnel to carry on the work with patients. To place upon the nursing school the responsibility for ward service is unfair to both patients and students.

An objection to the continuance of undergraduate nursing schools is the age at which students enter. The high school graduate usually begins her nursing education immediately after leaving high school at the age of eighteen. Adolescents of this immature age should not be in charge of psychiatric patients. They are not sufficiently stabilized emotionally to be placed in such a situation. The utilization of young and immature people for ward service is, in my opinion, a very questionable procedure.

For these reasons and others of more minor importance I believe that the interests of psychiatric patients would be best served by the discontinuance of the nursing schools for the education of general nurses and the substitution of other forms of nurse training.

School of Psychiatric Nursing. To meet the problem of mental nursing some hospitals and a few states have inaugurated a two-year course for psychiatric nurses. It is the contention of the proponents of this system that the mental hospital should concentrate upon the education of nurses for the specific field of psychiatry. They claim that the general nurse takes many courses that are unnecessary for one who is to care for mental patients and that two years' training in the techniques that are peculiarly applicable in the mental hospital is sufficient.

There are several reasons why this scheme is unsound and will probably not succeed. At a time when nursing leaders are emphasizing the necessity for better educated nurses, this is a definite step towards lowering standards. Psychiatry needs nurses with more training rather than less. The psychiatric nurse performs a more difficult and exacting task than any general nurse, and she should have correspondingly better educational equipment. Any specialty must be built on a foundation of general education and experience. Psychiatry is no exception to this rule. It is equivalent to the belief that psychiatrists do not need a general medical background but can get what special training they require in a shorter period of time. There can be no short cuts in either profession to the attainment of psychiatric skill and understanding.

Any educational scheme that is founded on the specific needs of a particular group of hospitals is not sound. When the institutions are saturated with the graduates from these schools, how will the others be absorbed? Without legal registration they can have no standing in the community. What would probably happen is that they would represent themselves as general nurses and add to an already overcrowded profession a group of poorly trained individuals who can reflect no credit on the institution which sponsored them.

Affiliate Nurse Education. There is a definite trend in nursing education to regard a course in theoretical and practical psychiatry as an essential part of general nurse training. When the movement reaches the point where a psychiatric course is essential to registration, the state hospitals will have to assume the burden of carrying on this instruction. It would be an excellent substitute for general nurse education. Such an undergraduate course should require at least four months and preferably be given during the second or third year. Both theoretical and practical instructions are essential. If the mental hospital is so situated that it is possible to give the lectures on psychiatry before the student actually enters upon her affiliation, the results will be more satisfactory. These lectures can be given either at the affiliating school or at the mental hospital if distance does not make it impossible. One session of two hours each week for a period of twelve weeks will cover the ground thoroughly, and when the students come to the institution their instruction consists of the application of this theory to the patient.

A suggested preliminary course is as follows:

Topical Outline of Affiliating Course

1. History of Mental Disorder
2. Mental Disease as a Public Health Problem
3. The Infection-Exhaustion Psychoses
4. The Toxic Psychoses
5. General Paresis
6. The Symptomatic Psychoses
7. Arteriosclerotic and Senile Psychoses
8. Borderline States
9. Manic-Depressive Psychoses
10. Schizophrenia
11. What is Mental Hygiene?
12. Mental Hygiene of Childhood
13. Mental Hygiene of Adolescence
14. The Human Personality

It will be noted that the introduction of the student to psychiatry is through the psychoses which have a direct physical causation. It is exceedingly difficult to lead her directly into the confusing mazes of manic-depressive or schizophrenic psychoses. This course should not be a mere recital of symptomatology but should seek to correlate and coördinate the mental mechanisms which accompany all disease. Unless this easy transition is deftly used we may find that the student is floundering about in a sea of vocabulary and misunderstood terminology. The simpler the course and the more gradually it develops from the physical to the highly complex psychological, the more successful it will be.

When the student enters the hospital for her practical work she follows her patients through in the same order. Her first service should be on the medical wards and the bedside instruction must be directed largely towards the relationship of the psyche and soma. From here she goes to the psychiatric wards, and finally to the admission ward, the outpatient clinic, and the child guidance clinic. Subsidiary services on which she has a service are hydrotherapy and occupational therapy. While this may seem to be a full program for a four months' course, only an introduction to psychiatry can be given, and if the student is guided intensively, it will give her at least a good orientation.

POSTGRADUATE EDUCATION

I am convinced that the great opportunity of the specialized hospital in the field of education is in postgraduate instruction. The mental institution can set up an educational system which is entirely divorced from ward responsibility, to which graduates of approved nursing schools may come for special courses that will fit them for the mental hospital service or general nursing. Such a plan would serve to attract well prepared graduate nurses to our service. Only candidates for this course should be accepted who have the proper educational background to appreciate and understand the significance of psychiatry, and no candidate should be accepted whose personality does not fit her for psychiatric nursing. Such a course should take at least nine months, to allow for a proper rotation of service.

As an example of a course for graduate students I offer the following:

AIMS

1. To sharpen the student's powers of observation.
2. To help her to interpret behavior.
3. To make constructive suggestions in the actual nursing care of the patient.
4. To understand the program of therapy and what part the nurse may play in it.
5. To appreciate the possibilities of prevention and the community aspects of the disease under discussion.

PSYCHIATRIC NURSING

I. *Overview*

"Education is the acquisition of the art of the utilization of knowledge."—Whitehead.[29] Like the proverbial people who can't see the forest for the trees, there are too many nurses who can't see the patients for the beds. Psychiatric nursing aims to correct this blind spot.

A. *Expectations for the Postgraduate Course*

1. *To educate nurses in psychiatry for the sake of the great numbers of patients who need special care.*
   a. Half the hospital beds in the country occupied by mental patients.
   b. Comparatively few nurses are taught psychiatry.
2. *To give nurses a better perspective on the whole field of nursing.*

   "The nursing arts must include the arts of health—as well as those of sick-nursing, and this includes the care of the mind as well as the body and group as well as individual nursing."—Stewart.[30]

   a. By understanding the mental and emotional complications in physical illness.

b. By recognizing incipient psychiatric disorders in hospital, home, and community.
c. By appreciating the importance of the influence of social factors (racial, religious, environmental.)

3. *To help nurses understand themselves.*
   a. Through the study of personalities.
      (1) Project: personality study—six months.
      (2) Mental health service as well as physical is offered.

B. *Methods*

"It seems clear that to have intelligent service it must be careful action based on intelligent understanding. Otherwise sooner or later significant symptoms are overlooked at some critical time. A proper discipline is conscientious acting on intelligent understanding."—W. H. Kilpatrick.[31]

1. The theoretical courses are designed to give the "intelligent understanding" of mental illness—its facts and opinions, its terminology and symptomatology, its social implication.
   a. An advantage of graduate courses is that they are all centered toward one main interest.
   b. Questions and criticisms are welcome.
2. Practical experience to teach "careful action."
   a. Hours on and off duty.
   b. Rotation of services.

II. *Description of Courses—First Semester*

A. *Psychiatry*

1. One-hour lectures weekly by staff members.
2. Two-hour conferences weekly conducted by lecturer, in which patient is discussed by students.

   "The purpose of the teaching method is to equip professional workers with a point of view as well as with body of knowledge which will enable them to coöperate with other professions toward a better understanding of the problems of human welfare. We are trying to integrate a mass of isolated facts and opinions with a concept of a human being suffering from the experience of a certain disease."—Leonard.[32]

B. *Psychology*—one hour weekly.

C. *Sociology*—two-hour period weekly.

Nursing is so essentially a socialized art that one must view patients not only as disease entities, or even as personalities, but as products of and members of society. Social health differs in accordance with the mores of the group. Mores are relative, but by understanding them we can appreciate the degree of social maladjustment present.

D. *Therapeutic Approaches*

III. *Points of Historical Interest*

IV. *Reading*

Bailey, Harriet—*Nursing Mental Diseases.* 3rd Edition.
Henderson & Gillespie—*Textbook of Psychiatry.*
Noyes, Arthur P.—*Textbook of Psychiatry.*
Annual Report of N.L.N.E. 1935—"Demonstration of a Method of Clinical Instruction." P. 161.
MacIver, Robert M.—*Contribution of Sociology to Social Work.*
Hart, Bernard—*Psychology of Insanity.*
Reminiscences of Linda Richards.

A. Project. Bibliography.

V. *Principles of Mental Nursing*

"The Hospital is a source of refuge for some, a means of protection to society in others, but above all a place where disordered minds may receive medical treatment that will help them find mental health." [33]

Objectivity.
Truthfulness.
Lack of Fear.
Individualized Care (hyper- and hypo-activity).
Occupations for Mind and Body.
Supportive Care.

Feeding—elimination—bathing—exercise—sleep.
See articles on "Sedatives" in *American Journal of Nursing.*[34, 35]
Responsibilities as a Teacher.

VI. *Precautions*

See *Manual* and Ward Routine Books of Worcester State Hospital.

Locked doors, instrument and silver counts, fire rules, accidents, suicides.

PSYCHIATRIC NURSING

VII. *Terminology*

Bailey—Glossary in *Nursing Mental Diseases.*

Project: Patients who exhibit certain symptoms, with examples of behavior.

VIII. *Tube-Feeding*

Indications for—
Equipment—
Formulae—
Method of giving—dangers involved.
Detailed care of feeding problems.

IX. *Care of Patients with Alcoholic Psychoses*

X. *Encephalogram*

A. Preparation of patient.
B. Tray set-up—sterile, unsterile.

OUTLINE FOR WEEKLY SYMPOSIUM

I. *The Disease Process*

Historical background — etiology — pathology — symtomatology—treatment—prognosis—epidemiology.

II. *The Patient*

Heredity—pre-psychotic personality (body-type, mood, intelligence, character)—course of present illness —predisposing factors—typical and atypical symptoms —mental status—behavior—reasons for admission to hospital.

$$\frac{\text{CC.} \quad \text{P.I.}}{\text{P.H.}}$$

III. *Social Aspects*

Home environment—racial, religious, family, economic factors with the problems involved—recommendations for follow-up care—social agencies available—possibilities for re-education in the home.

IV. *Nursing Care*

Patient's physical condition and treatment thereof—eating and sleeping habits—cleanliness—coöperation toward routine—special nursing problems called forth by patient's behavior.

N.B. This is considered the most important part of the discussion and should sum up points emphasized under other headings. We are primarily interested in *nursing* the patient.

PROJECTS

I. *Bibliography*

Textbooks, reference books, articles, fiction, biography. Give publisher and date of publication and make appropriate comments on each item.

II. *Definitions of terms used.*

III. *Personality Study*

Has psychiatric nursing helped or hindered in self-analysis and understanding? Be as specific or as general as you wish but be honest.

IV. Applications of the principles of psychiatric nursing in general hospitals to pediatric nursing, to public health nursing, and to private duty nursing.

V. Outline a mental hygiene program for schools of nursing for the students themselves and for the more intelligent nursing of the patients.

VI. *Book Reviews*

Choose a book, either fiction or biography, which seems to exemplify some mental or emotional aberration. Describe the mechanisms involved and theorize about possible adjustments.

Suggestions:	*The Folks*	by Ruth Suckow
	The Locomotive God	" W. E. Leonard
	The Idiot	" Dostoievsky
	The World Outside	" Hans Fallada
	Giants in the Earth	" O. E. Rolvaag

PRACTICAL EXPERIENCE

Admission of Patient
Discharge of Patient

Feeding of Patient—
cafeteria—spoon-feeding—tube-feeding.

Baths—
ward baths—admission bath—bath house—continuous tubs.

Packs—
wet sheet pack—restraining sheet—figures of eight.

Physiotherapy—
diathermy.

Operating room—
luetic clinic.

Therapy—
O.T.—farm—walking—entertainments—ward games.

Medications—
oral—subcutaneous—rectal.

HEAD NURSES

Education of personnel should not be allowed to lapse after the employee has entered the service. Though we are able to raise the requirements for entrance into the service, instruction should continue if the nurse is to grow in mental calibre and be of real value. At least one course each year should be given to head nurses in addition to the one they receive when they enter the hospital. As an example of such a course the following has been tried:

COURSE FOR HEAD NURSES

1. *Public Relationships.* The importance of the relative in psychiatry cannot be over-emphasized. The relationship with the general public is one of the aspects of hospital psychiatry that the nurse should understand.

2. *The Importance of Psychiatric Nursing Records.* If the observations of the nurse are to be of value to the psychiatrist, she must be taught how to make them worth while.

3. *The Ward Routine.* Administration of a psychiatric ward requires considerable managerial ability. Ward management is very essential in such a course.

4. *Psychotherapy.* If the nurse is not to undo everything the psychiatrist is trying to accomplish, she must have instruction.

5. *Psychiatric Research.* Head nurses should be informed of the research that is being carried on in psychiatry and encouraged to develop a research attitude towards their own problems. It is upon their techniques that the research worker depends for his data.

6. *Occupational Therapy.* The nurse should have a comprehensive knowledge of this most important therapeutic weapon.

7. *Hydrotherapy.* Special instruction in hydrotherapy should be given every head nurse. This should be both theoretical and practical.

8. *Recreational Program.* Ward recreation is an important part of psychiatric nursing. The organization of patients in play is an indispensable part of her responsibility.

9. *Preventive Psychiatry.* The nurse is an important factor in the mental hygiene program of the hospital. She should have training in the clinics attached to the hospital.

10. *Inspection Trips to Other Institutions.* Nurses should have an opportunity to visit jails, almshouses, orphanages, and similar institutions as a part of their psychiatric education.

Nurse Supervisors

An advanced course for supervisors, dealing with psychiatry and psychiatric administration, should be a regular part of the educational activities. This would consist of a weekly seminar presided over by the superintendent, assistant superintendent, or clinical director. The regular session should be supplemented by frequent ward walks for the demonstration of cases and daily conferences with the director of nursing for the discussion of practical hospital matters. The following course would be indicated for such a group:

1. *The Supervisor as a Leader.* Discussion of types of leadership and the qualities necessary for nursing leaders.

2. *Building Morale in the Group.* Deals with the practical methods by which a group spirit may be inculcated in the ward personnel.

3. *The Goal of the Hospital.* A discussion of practical methods by which the hospital goal may be achieved.

4. *Fundamental Motivations Behind Human Conduct.* A discussion dealing with the inborn tendencies which cause conduct, reflex action, instinctive behavior, and the guidance and control of instincts. This is in the light of practical personnel and patient problems as they are presented.

5. *The Use and Control of Emotions.* Personnel and patient problems with reference to such emotions as fear, anger, and hatred.

6. *Individual and Group Habits.* Habit formation is as important in the group as it is in the individual. Organization problems in the light of habit formation present a new aspect.

7. *Will and Personality.* Might include personality studies. The discussion covers the types of personalities and the probable cause of them.

8. *Defense Mechanisms.* How do both patient and employee use these to avoid unpleasant situations?

9. *Hospital Pedagogy.* The importance of teaching and instructing new employees is stressed and methods of carrying out the principles are discussed.

10. *Standards of Performance.* Administrative checks are necessary for the estimation of the value of an employee to the organization. A discussion of methods to accomplish this purpose.

11. *Methods of Handling People.* There are techniques of administration that should be learned by those who direct the activities of others.

12. *Personal Efficiency.* A discussion of the proper division of time, the psychology of neatness, etc.

ATTENDANTS

A course for attendants should be practical and given in simple, non-technical language. It must be devised to enable the individual to apply the material to his daily work. Such a course is the following:

COURSE FOR ATTENDANTS

I.	Orientation Series	6 hours
II.	Laboratory—Necessity for	1 hour
III.	Hospital Housekeeping	2 hours

IV.	Routine Reports	1 hour
V.	Practical Nursing	16 hours
VI.	Hospital Routine	4 hours
VII.	Hydrotherapy	4 hours
VIII.	O. T.	2 hours
		36 hours

OUTLINE OF COURSE

I. Orientation
  1. Introduction
    a. Objectives of the course
    b. Mental disease a public health problem
    c. Massachusetts' solution of the problem of mental disease
    d. The individual's place in the state hospital program
  2. Tour of the Hospital
    a. Operating Room Suite
    b. Radio Room
    c. Medical Library
    d. Patients' Library
    e. Steward's Department
    f. Kitchens
    g. Boiler Room
    h. Laboratory
  3. Relation of Hospital to Community
    a. Research
    b. Child Guidance
    c. Types of Commitment
  4. Discussion of the Manual for Ward Employees
    a. Fire Regulations
  5. The Philosophy of the Physician
  6. Something of the background and history of the care of the mentally ill
    a. Misconceptions that have been our heritage and the facts which refute them
    b. General attitudes of approach to mental patients

II. Laboratory
  1. Use
  2. Procedures for specimens

III. Hospital Housekeeping
  1. Repairs
  2. Conservation of hospital supplies
  3. Airing needs
  4. Care of mattresses
  5. Prevention of bedbugs—roaches
  6. Laundry

IV. Routine Charts
  1. Ward reports—night reports—accident slips—restraint and seclusion slips—admission records—mortuary slips.

V. Practical Nursing
  1. Bed-making
    a. Standing bed—occupied bed
    b. Ether bed
  2. Bed bath
    a. Lifting of patients
    b. A.M. and P.M. care (alcohol rub, brushing teeth, combing hair)
  3. T.P.R. (Temperature, Pulse, and Respiration)
  4. Pressure sores
    a. Cause
    b. Precaution
    c. Care of
  5. Enemas
  6. Pediculi
    a. Treatment
    b. Use of durbac comb—Head—Body
  7. Hot and Cold Applications
    a. Hot water bottles
    b. Ice caps
  8. Symptoms to Observe and Report
    a. Loss of Weight
    b. Appetite
    c. Cough
    d. Sores
    e. Eruptions
  9. Care of Body after Death
    a. Preparation
    b. Visit to morgue

c. Use of refrigerator
d. Courtesy to relatives of patients on D.L.

10. Admission of patient to hospital
    a. Routine carried out
    b. Record
    c. Care of valuables, clothing, teeth, and glasses
11. Emergencies
    a. Hanging
    b. Choking
    c. Clothing afire
    d. Fainting
    e. Fractures
    f. Wounds
    g. Bruises
    h. Foreign bodies in ears, nose, eyes
12. Nursing Care of Excited Patients
    a. Proper and improper method of handling
    b. Deteriorated patients
    c. Feeding problems
    d. Seizures
    e. Old people
    f. Depressions
13. Preparation for Tube-Feeding

VI. Hospital Routine
1. Purpose of locked doors
2. Escapes—prevention, seriousness of fire drill routine
3. Actual fires—Employees' responsibility
4. Clinics—Procedure for assembling
5. Cafeteria—Duties while on duty there
6. Entertainments
7. Suicidal precautions—meaning

VII. Hydrotherapy—Lectures
1. Wet sheet pack—Continuous bath—Tonic baths
2. When assigned to Hydrotherapy Department, attendant is under direct supervision of Hydrotherapist

VIII. O.T.
1. Application of theory under supervision of graduate in charge of ward
2. Types of Therapy which can be used by attendants with Doctors' orders

3. Recreation
4. Beauty Parlor
5. Letter-writing
6. Barber Shops

PROFESSIONAL STAFF

A course in advanced psychiatry is a necessity for staff members below the grade of senior. This statement is only applicable to the hospital that requires at least one year of psychiatric experience before staff appointment. For the institution which requires no previous training in psychiatry the course will be more elemental. The following topical outline is offered as being suitable for this purpose:

Course for Junior Professional Staff

1. Classification of Mental Diseases
2. Biometrical Approach to Mental Disease
3. Freudian Mechanisms
4. Theory of Kretschmer
5. Sociological Approach
6. The Contribution of Psychology
7. Psychometry
8. The Endocrine Glands in Mental Disease
9. Psychosomatic Relationships
10. Place of the Laboratory
11. Child Guidance
12. Contribution of Social Service

Seminars dealing with administration in its broadest sense should be conducted by the superintendent. These are attended by the entire professional staff. A topical outline of such seminars is offered:

Course in Administration

1. Laws Regulating Deportation
2. The Narcotic Law
3. Analysis of State Laws Dealing with Mental Disease
4. Regulations of the Control Body
5. State Medicine
6. Future of the Mental Hospital

7. Local Social Administration
8. Statistics of Mental Disease
9. Importance of the Family in Psychiatry
10. Psychiatry in Medical Education
11. Organization of Mental Hospital Clinics
12. Public Education

It should not be understood that any one individual gives all these courses. The clinical director arranges for the leader of each seminar and guides him in the selection of material to be presented. They should be scheduled in advance with a bibliography in order that those attending may be prepared for free discussion.

Lay Employees

Formal seminars are not practicable for this group. Each member, as he enters the service, should be required to take the orientation course. Education must be carried on through department heads. I am convinced that more technical education dealing with the particular kind of work the individual is doing would be of tremendous benefit to the State hospitals. The salaries paid to cooks, laundry workers, and farm employees are rarely equal to those paid by the community for similar work. Therefore the hospital does not attract the best trained and experienced individual. It becomes necessary for the hospital to offer an opportunity to prepare for advancement to make up for the deficiency in pay. A course for laundry washers dealing with the fundamental facts of washing processes met with an enthusiastic reception by the workers. It covered the simple chemistry of water, the mechanical action of the washwheel, the chemical reaction of clothing to various types of washing powders and soaps, methods of testing the performance of the process, and a consideration of formulas. The result of this course was a marked improvement in the quality of laundry work and a better spirit among the workers. Similar courses for cooks and farm workers would be valuable.

STUDENTS FROM OUTSIDE HOSPITAL

Undergraduate Teaching. This is a clinical clerkship for senior medical students. They are assigned to the hospital for one month. Undergraduates are frequently utilized by mental institutions during the summer vacation period. Whatever time is spent, the hospital is responsible for making it a real teaching experience and it should be largely clinical.

1. *Major Case Assignments.* Each student studies two patients during his month of residence. Newly admitted patients with physical disease are assigned because students are more at ease in a general hospital environment. Special medical interests are always kept in mind. A case of post-operative psychosis is given to the man who is interested in surgery. If he leans towards obstetrics a puerperal case is selected.

The student is responsible for the following studies:

1. Physical Examination
   (checked by internist)
2. Psychiatric and Medical History
   (checked by social worker and psychiatrist)
3. Mental Status
   (checked by psychiatrist in charge of service)
4. Progress Notes
   a. Somatic Status
   b. Mental Observations
5. Diagnostic Summary
   (checked by psychiatrist in charge of service)
6. Complete and Detailed Therapeutic Program
   (checked by clinical director)

2. *Minor Case Assignments. Continued Treatment Patients.* From six to eight patients of the continued treatment group are assigned to each student. These are usually cases that have been studied by other students from the same school.

Students hand in summaries to two of these cases each week after reading the record and interviewing the patient. These are checked by the clinical director.

3. *Ward Walks and Interviews.* These are held daily by the intermediate and senior staff. They are devoted to a discussion

of the major case assignments. Statistical diagnosis is rarely mentioned. Every effort is made to have the student get the idea that the diagnostic label is only of statistical importance and that rapport and a thorough study of the patient are the fundamental things. Discussions on psychotherapy occupy an important rôle in these ward walks.

4. *Assigned Reading.* Few textbooks are used except for reference. Journal assignments are made to each student and he is expected to select articles that appeal to him. He makes a written report, giving journal, title, name of author, and a brief abstract. Each student must make 25 abstracts during his month of service, and weekly conferences are held to check this assignment. Students are acquainted with the major contribution to psychiatric literature and they learn to use a medical library.

5. *Staff Conferences.* Each student must present one case before the staff. This is valuable experience. It helps him to organize his thinking and develop poise and ease in presenting cases.

6. *Psychiatric Histories.* The chief social worker instructs the student in the technique of securing a psychiatric-social history.

7. *Clinico-Pathological Conference.* This is a monthly staff meeting at which an autopsied case is presented by the psychiatrist, internist, and pathologist. Attendance at this conference is compulsory.

8. *Luetic Clinics.* The technique of lumbar punctures and the administration of intravenous therapy is taught to the students.

9. *Child Guidance Clinic.* A conference led by the clinic director. Discussion centers around the type of cases and methods of treatment.

10. *Patients' Relatives* (Major Cases). Students contact the relatives of their major assignments under the direction of the senior psychiatrist.

11. *Legal Considerations.* One conference is devoted to a discussion of the legal implications of the psychoses, including the commitment laws.

12. *Home Visits.* Where possible the students make one

visit to the home of a patient in company with a social worker.

13. *Reports to Schools.* After the student has completed his assigned period at the hospital a report is sent to the school giving the following information:

1. Attitude towards his experience
2. Technical ability
3. Aptitude for medical work
4. Personality

Graduate Internes. Graduates who are interested in a psychiatric internship come for one of three reasons. A few who do not intend to adopt psychiatry as a specialty see the necessity of a well-rounded training. After completing a general internship they devote a year to psychiatry. A larger group accept psychiatric internships because they wish to specialize in psychiatry. The third group is made up of internes from general hospitals whose term includes a four months' residence in the psychiatric hospital.

It is to be hoped that these graduate internes will increase in number, and they undoubtedly will if mental hospitals will organize to give the proper instruction. A rotating service is an important consideration for graduates.

1. Male Psychiatric Service
2. Female Psychiatric Service
3. Medical Service
4. Research Service
5. Child Guidance Clinic.

Carefully thought out courses of instruction for each group of students are requisite for such an educational program. Students cannot be exploited but must be given something that will repay them for the financial sacrifice they make when they take the course. It is the exceptional student who does not more than repay the institution in actual work performed. They become very valuable after their preliminary training has been completed and are capable of doing a great deal of routine work and carrying some responsibility. No student should receive any salary beyond maintenance. To pay anyone to take an education indicates that the educational offering is not very valuable.

I freely admit that an educational plan in a mental hospital means sacrifice in time and money. I insist that the hospital has a responsibility in this field and must, sooner or later, prepare to carry out that responsibility. The rewards that come are the satisfaction and stimulation that educational efforts inevitably create, and the addition to the hospital personnel of a group of inquisitive, active, knowledge-seeking individuals. The patient on the ward invariably reaps the benefit of these activities.

Chapter 11

COÖRDINATED RESEARCH

For a hundred years state governments have tried to stem the ever-increasing tide of mental disease by intermittent and frantic scrambles to provide more housing accommodations. Even this policy has not been pursued with any intelligent consistency. In only a few states has there been any concerted effort to study the problem in a broad way and inaugurate a sound program of construction in accordance with the findings of such a comprehensive survey. Few states have adequate statistical departments that are capable of guiding legislators in their attempts to keep abreast of the public needs. As a result, an attitude of pessimism or indifference has entered into the situation. Many states have not even carried out their responsibilities in building during the past five years. Economic conditions have interfered with such programs as were in operation. Overcrowding has become acute because of the cessation of building. Budgets have been drastically reduced and relatively little could be used for construction. The entire scheme of meeting this problem of mental disease has been completely upset in many states.

It would seem to be an opportune time to pause and study the situation. Is there not some other method of approach which gives promise of eventually reducing the burden? As has been pointed out in another chapter, a state may adopt a parsimonious policy which will bring immediate savings but which will cost more eventually, or it may meet the problem in a constructive way by increasing present costs with the hope of effecting greater saving in the future. Every state is confronted with the necessity of choosing between these two policies, and the choice will frequently be the result of the educational efforts of hospital and community psychiatrists. We may not be able to change the attitude and thinking of legislators over-night, but a quiet, persistent emphasis upon other approaches will finally turn the tide towards a more constructive attitude.

What have we to offer the state as a partial substitute for a program of building to increase bed capacity? One way is to increase the amount of psychiatric research going on. If we could put up with the problem of overcrowding for a few years longer and utilize a portion of the funds that would be put into building for the inauguration of a coördinated attack upon the psychoses, the result twenty-five years from now would be astounding.

The victims of mental disorder represent a tremendous and wasteful leak in our social system. It is a foolish dissipation of man-power to permit this to continue decade after decade and give no thought to it except to house the product of the leakage. A long-time, carefully considered policy of investigation into the causation of mental disease would undoubtedly bring results in prevention and cure. Research efforts can be computed in terms of actual money. Perhaps the most outstanding example of the rewards of psychiatric research is general paresis. Early psychiatrists had no knowledge as to the exact cause of the disease. They attributed it to all kinds of misconduct and dissipation. But the one thing they agreed upon was the fatal termination. With few exceptions, victims of general paresis died within three years. Quiet, persistent investigation over a long period of years culminated in a demonstration of the spirochete in the brains of paretics, and syphilis was established as the one and only cause of general paresis. From this beginning, therapeutic efforts progressed rapidly, and the mental hospital which is actually treating these patients has a discharge rate of from 35 per cent to 45 per cent of those admitted. We look forward confidently to even greater triumphs in the handling of this particular disorder. Does research pay?

The industrialist does not hesitate to pour great sums of money into commercial investigation because he knows that it will bring him rich returns. He is certain that, given brains and money, research will sooner or later solve every problem for him.

Psychiatric research has been shockingly neglected in the past. It is true that individual efforts have been directed towards a solution of some of our problems, but most of these individuals have worked against great odds. They have met indifference, opposition, lack of funds, and the superiority of a traditional attitude. But in spite of resistance, they have given the fruits of their labor to those who have rendered so little assistance. All honor to these hardy pioneers in psychiatric research.

What is the reason for the neglect of research in this field? Perhaps one of the most important factors is the enormous complexity of the problem. We are dealing with reactions that are so subtle and many-sided that it is difficult to know where to begin. We do not even know what the disease is that we are studying, except on a purely descriptive level. Because of this, all investigative efforts have been built around isolated variables which in only a few instances have led to results. Individual research is practically always limited to isolated functions. In order to see processes in their relationships—which is the real object of research—many aspects of the problem must be investigated on the same experimental subject. In psychiatry coöperative investigation is almost a necessity.

A mass attack on the psychoses will eventually bring results in a better understanding of causation. When a research team consisting of psychiatrist, chemist, internist, psychologist, physicist, sociologist, social worker, and administrator studies the same patient, each from his particular angle, and when such teams are multiplied a hundred times, we shall then begin to make a real contribution to our understanding of the psychoses.

Why should research be carried on in mental hospitals? There are many reasons why the hospital with a large patient population is, under certain conditions, an ideal place to carry on such investigations. Research is a costly process even when carried on as economically as possible. When new plants must be constructed and maintained, the cost becomes almost prohibitive. The hospital is already in existence and functioning. The plant is there, the maintenance is provided for, and the patients are in residence. We have the theater, the stage setting, and the company. All that is needed is the play, the director, and some stars. Philanthropic organizations are recognizing the economy of research when conducted in existing concerns and are subsidizing such arrangements rather than putting their money into new projects.

The psychoses cannot be studied without psychotic patients. Hospitals have large populations of mental patients who live under controlled conditions and remain for long periods of time. This clinical material should be an important factor in attracting research workers.

In State systems there exists an opportunity for coördination which is impossible when isolated units are working. The Psychiatric Institute furnishes research leadership for the entire psychiatric group. Such coördination prevents duplication of effort and waste of money.

The contact of the research worker with the actual, everyday problems of the hospital has a stabilizing influence on his thinking. It keeps him in reality. Usually investigators tend to become cloistered and get too far away from the practical side of the problem.

Organization of Hospital Research

Research can be carried on successfully only in a friendly atmosphere. It must be an integral part of the organization and must be accepted by the entire group as a worthwhile project. Much of this spirit is stimulated by the superintendent. If he believes that the hospital should participate in such a program and is willing to make sacrifices to carry it on, the proper spirit will soon be created. The doubting Thomas in the professional group will either change his attitude or be eliminated. But without the whole-hearted and enthusiastic coöperation of the administration, research dies rapidly. The administrator need not necessarily be familiar with investigative techniques, but he must have the spirit of research strongly developed within him.

Director of Research

Experimental activities will never be profitable as long as they are a by-product of the hospital routine. While small investigations can and should be carried on in the daily work, the profitable approach to the problems of psychiatry is a systematic and orderly procedure under the direction of one man who can give his entire time to the work. Research calls for special qualifications of personality and technical proficiency which everyone does not possess. The characteristics which make a research worker may prevent his being an efficient ward psychiatrist. The mere desire to investigate a problem does not necessarily mean that the individual is a competent investigator. In addition to this he must have some interest in the problem of the psychoses and the contribution he can make through his particular approach. It is not always possible to make a competent research worker out of a good psychiatrist or a good chemist. He must, in addition, have that particular type of thinking which we call "research-minded." What are the essential traits of a research worker aside from technical proficiency? He must possess a controlled and subordinated curiosity to the aims of science, curiosity that impels him to get at the underlying reasons back of all phenomena. He should have imagination. This trait must be under strict control, else he becomes a mere visionary or an arm-chair day-dreamer. He should have great respect for the magnitude of the problem in which he is interested and not under-estimate the difficulties or over-estimate his own abilities. He must have a sincere conviction of the insufficiency of his knowledge and approach all problems in a humble spirit. He should be willing to gain additional knowledge where and from whom he can. Workers who are satisfied to dangle their legs from the heights of their specialties and keep their heads in the clouds of professional arrogance may be in a position which is very satisfying to themselves, but they do not contribute much to a coöperative research. But in spite of this humble spirit, the true research worker has self-confidence and great courage. Without these traits he becomes a vacillating, unstable, and unreliable individual.

The director, in addition to these qualities, must have a certain amount of administrative ability in order to coördinate the activities. Unless he can do this we may have projects being carried on without relation to each other or to the main idea. I am not unmindful of the rugged individualism of the research worker. He is apt to resent dictation, or what he is pleased to call regimentation. He is a lone wolf and rarely does he run with the pack. But in spite of this characteristic, it is possible to give freedom in the selection of projects and methodology and at the same time keep the program from wandering off into blind alleys.

The director should be a psychiatrist but he must be a broad-gauged one with the type of training and personality that will attract men to work under his leadership. A combined research, which seems to be the indicated mode of attack upon the problems of psychiatry, must be thought of as personified in a super-human scientist. To such a scientist a discipline is a method and it is essential that he choose that method which is suited to the problem and not let a predilection for a particular discipline dictate his problem. The director of research is the integrating force of this super-human animal which consists of many parts. This requires one trait above all others—objectivity. If he can reach that objectivity he can direct the various talents of his research group into a performance that creates the impression of coming from a superhuman polyhistor. The director is the pivotal point around which any research group is built, and the administrator who wishes to create such a department will do well to consider carefully the individual who will direct the work. There are distressingly few men in the world who meet all the requirements, but young men are being trained and will be available as rapidly as proper positions can be found for them.

A word of warning should be injected at this point. The administrator who becomes enthusiastic and says, "Let's do research," without thinking the project through, is due for some bitter disappointments. And this, in my opinion, is one of the great dangers of an extensive program. No man should be permitted to work on any research project until he has thought out every step of his approach. And by the same token, no administrator should rush headlong into such a program without giving careful thought to the sacrifices it requires and where it may lead. Merely puttering will get us nowhere. Both desire and planning must precede action. But one cannot prevent the "research-minded" individual from carrying on critical investigations any more than one can keep the artist from painting a picture or the musician from composing music. It is an expression of the inner self and cannot be dammed up by obstacles. The individual who gives up because he does not find everything to his liking probably should not be a research worker. He will do better in some other line of activity.

A research board made up of individuals who have had experience in investigative work is of great assistance to the administrator who wishes to organize a research department. Such a board or committee is composed of men who, while they may not have a working knowledge of the problems of psychiatry, do understand the general principles of research.

Individual workers must be required to work out complete plans for any project in which they are interested and the protocol should be carefully checked and approved by the research board or committee. The following outline is used by the Massachusetts Research Committee which is a part of the Department of Mental Diseases:

OUTLINE OF POINTS TO BE COVERED IN ANY PROTOCOL

Project: Complete title should be given with particular care that it presents a complete story of the study to be pursued.

Rationale: Here we need an orientation of the problem. What is the particular problem that suggests itself? Why is it worth studying? How is it best to approach the problem? Is it a check on similar investigations or does it cover a gap in our present knowledge?

Bibliography: It is essential that all literature pertaining to the problem be reviewed and every protocol must have a complete bibliography. Duplication of work is wasteful.

Procedure: We have the problem before us. Now what is the best way of procedure in obtaining the answers to our problem? What are the methods to be used? What types of patients will be needed? What materials, instruments, and personnel will be necessary? What are the various steps to be followed? Is this order of procedure the best one that can be evolved?

Controls: If the proposed research project is not to descend to the level of mere description, then a concerted effort must be made to establish suitable controls. Inasmuch as the controls in each study will vary in accordance with the type of study, it is not practicable to outline this further.

Sources of Error: A few of the factors are listed which have been found to be of importance in various projects. Of course other sources of error will be noted in different studies and it may be that the following will not apply to any specific problem. Every project carries its own pitfalls. Search for them *before* you begin.

1. It is wise to make an effort to reduce all variables so that in the selection of patients we have a group which is sufficiently alike to render some meaning to our study of a single variable.
2. Look for conditions which might modify the results and see that they are controlled or eliminated.
3. When observations are made on patients, see that the same time of day is used and particularly the same interval after meals.
4. Check differences in age and physical characteristics of both patients and controls.
5. Temperature and humidity of room in which observations are made should be kept uniform.
6. See that patients and controls are free from chronic disease. It is of little use to conduct an experiment on drugs affecting the circulation, for example, if we are dealing with patients with cardiovascular disease.
7. It is advisable to have observations made by the same person or by similarly trained persons.
8. Variations in technique between laboratories are common. If we wish a certain result we should see that the same technique is used and in one laboratory, with the same personnel doing the work on repeated examinations. This will cut down the laboratory error which is always a problem.
9. Include as large a number of cases as is feasible. Small samples mean greater chance variation and lessen the significance of findings. One study based on a large number of cases is worth several small ones.

Records: Records and methods of recording on the part of observers should be rigidly standardized. The method of recording, time, etc., should be meticulously outlined. Notes should be made recording the reactions of patients to the procedure. All recording should be done immediately following the observation and should never be trusted to memory.

Time Required: An estimate should be made of the time which will be required for the completion of the experiment. Research projects should not drag on indefinitely but should be conducted in accordance with a definite schedule of operations. It is well to include plans for the writing, revisions, and publication of the material.

Expenses: It is highly advisable that some estimate be made of the cost of materials and personnel required for the proposed project. In some cases the purchase of expensive equipment for a single experiment will not be found advisable. In other cases the end results of the study will not justify the expenditure. In others it may be possible to select certain projects which can be completed on limited expenditures, particularly where funds are not too plentiful. Results will usually bring additional funds. It is well to estimate the cost of your project before beginning, otherwise it may have to be discontinued after much time and money have been spent.

Furthermore, every research project must have an aim. In a recent issue of *Philosophy of Science* John Somerville [36] discusses the "Forgotten Problem." By this he means the "aims of science." He points out that everybody is debating methods but nobody speaks of aims. A method is not a thing in itself but should be subordinated to the aims it serves. Therefore, before the director and administrator decide upon methods of approach, they should carefully think out the aims of the research and fit into the scheme those representatives of disciplines or methods which will best contribute to the accomplishment of the general aim. It requires great force of character to withstand the pressure which leads one into unprofitable by-paths. An individual who has acquired great skill in a particular technique may be brought into the group for the specific purpose of working with a particular problem in which his method is indicated. But disaster comes if after the accomplishment of the specific problem he is kept on and allowed to set up new projects because his methods can handle them.

DEPARTMENTALIZATION

In a joint research, which is probably the best approach to psychiatric problems, departmentalization is inevitable after the project has reached a certain point. A certain amount of regimentation is essential for financial reasons even before scientific considerations are taken into account. Individual research is possible only when each worker is able to raise the funds necessary for his work privately. To have the financial security which comes with a common fund, the worker must make certain sacrifices in the interest of the common aim of the research. To distribute such funds as are available there must be a central organ or control body which makes the decision as to the allotment to each worker. The greatest sacrifice the worker must make in a situation of this kind is that the project upon which he works will not be wholly his. Investigations must be interlocking in order that all may profit by them. The principle of regimentation must be accepted by every worker who comes into such an organization. It is not the principle but the way it is carried out that may render it objectionable.

The administrator who seeks to build a research group in his organization will select a director. If the project is simple, one person can probably carry it out. But what psychiatric problem is simple? As the project becomes more complex, the director will require assistants or advisors in many fields. He will need internists, biochemists, psychologists, sociologists, and biometricians. Each of these assistants will, in time, have more to do than they can accomplish alone and assistants must be hired. And then we have departmentalization and the real troubles of the administrator begin. Department heads devise the procedures on which assistants are working and are responsible to the director for results. A certain amount of authority is therefore indispensable for the department head. Hence regimentation in a joint research cannot be avoided.

The ideal way of carrying on this type of organization is through the principle of participative democracy which has been advocated throughout the pages of this book. The selection of research problems can be used as an illustration. In a completely regimented organization the problem would be assigned by the director to an assistant and the latter would work it out. But this is the kind of monarchal organization to which the worker rightfully objects. The proposal of the project should come from the assistant, and one who does not have the imagination to propose his own projects should not be retained in any research group no matter what his paper qualifications are. Financial resources for research are too limited to waste money on sterile and unproductive individuals. And the administrator who is tempted to retain men in a research for sentimental reasons had better not embark on a venture of this kind.

All proposed protocols should be submitted to a committee consisting of the director and at least three department heads, appointed for the specific purpose of examining the project and passing upon its feasibility. The project outline should be submitted, in writing, to all members of the committee and they should be given at least two weeks to state their comments, in writing. These comments are addressed to the chairman of the committee, who would summarize them and present the summary to the group, at a meeting. The deviser of the project should be present. Changes and modifications would be made or the project rejected entirely, the reasons being given. No project should ever be put into operation without passing through such a committee. No research worker should be exempt from this requirement. Research workers may feel that such a procedure is an insult to their prestige. But the administrator who must furnish the funds is entitled to know what is going on, even if he is not always in a position to criticize a highly specialized project.

The influence of this committee should be far-reaching and even the director should not put into operation a project to which the majority of the committee takes exception or accept it in a form to which the majority of the committee objects. The committee is as responsible for the project as the man who submits it.

Assignment of problems is at times unavoidable in a joint research. A worker may have a valuable idea which can best be carried on by a man in another field. Such assignments are legitimate if certain conditions are observed:

1. The problem must be approved by the committee.
2. The worker to whom the problem is to be assigned should be a member of the committee.
3. The problem must suit the field of interest and technical training of the assignee.
4. The project should not interfere with the regular work on which the assignee is engaged.

One of the dangers of any research is the temptation to keep on with the compilation of data after the need of further material diminishes. The "terminal facilities" of research workers are not, as a rule, well developed. When the project fails, the originator frequently tries to explain away this failure to himself. He may even try to force results. In good projects the worker may acquire some kind of rhythm and be unable to stop. This is not for the best interest of either worker or organization. The director should be prepared to stop any project when it ceases to be profitable, but always in conference with the worker.

Research workers should not be permitted to accumulate data without digesting them and relating them to the general aim of the research. The worker who wants to go on year after year, piling up information without being required to give any account of what he is doing, has no place in a coöperative research. He should be required at regular intervals to report progress on his project. This report would preferably go to the problem committee for scrutiny.

Coöperation in Research

This is a much overworked word but capable of as many interpretations as there are people using it. Some believe that it is a trick machine which the administration should supply and operate and out of which the synthesis of research should drop, wrapped in cellophane. Others seem to feel that coöperation means that someone else should do all the work. Another group sees in it the acceptance of all the ideas and desires of the one who uses the term.

Coöperation is neither a fantastic nor a preposterous proposition. It is not obtrusive, neither does it advertise itself. Coöperation goes on in some form continuously and unconsciously in science. The fact that research workers publish their results and make their data available to others is an act of coöperation. The administration can hasten or inhibit coöperation but cannot compel it. The director and administrator can initiate it by choosing the right kind of men, through setting an example by invoking coöperation in their own projects, and through unobtrusive infiltration of the doctrine. Every man in the organization is responsible for the actual operation of true coördination. Each man must make it his duty to work himself into the understanding of the results of his co-workers in all fields of the research. The internist should not simply file away the reprints of psychological articles but he should overcome the limitations of his training and he should—he *must*—understand them. Once he has understood them, he should attempt to translate the findings in terms of organic physiology and pathology. He should attempt to verify the physiological implications and to evaluate them as to the significance of his own findings. Conversely, psychologists and psychiatrists should become intimately familiar with the organic findings and try to understand their psychological correlates. This is coöperative research. It is the secret of one project growing out of another and the "interlocking" of projects. Constant consultation and interchange of ideas among workers is essential in this kind of research.

The administrator must insist that workers regard this type of coöperation as their duty. Their merits should not be judged only on the basis of published results but also on the fact of whether or not they have attempted to and are able to carry out the desired functions of coöperation. It should be a principle that research men are paid for producing work in their own field but also for integrating their work into other fields.

The Editorial Board

All research results require confirmation, checking, and discussion by co-workers in other organizations. In view of this fact, publications should be reviewed by the hospital editorial board, which will have the authority to demand that statements emanating from quantitative findings be strictly in accord with the data. Qualitative opinions, however, should be entirely on the responsibility of the author, although the board should offer friendly criticism on this point. It should have the right to veto in case the paper is discreditable. The membership of this board will vary with the local situation but should include the superintendent of the hospital and the director of research.

It is to be expected that each research investigation will have by-products, and these should not be retained for presentation with the main paper but should be published separately and as early as possible. Workers who save all the aspects of their work for one publication usually defeat their own purpose. Such a procedure results in cluttering up the paper, obscuring the main issue, and devaluating the by-products. The administrator has a right to expect a major paper from every research worker, a publication every twelve to eighteen months. It is understood that research should not be carried on simply for the purpose of publishing papers, but publications presumably are the digested results of data that have been accumulated. They represent the checks that the worker is making on his own research.

SELECTION OF RESEARCH WORKERS

There are certain principles that should govern the selection of the heads of departments in a coördinated research project. As a first consideration the administrator should insist that, as a requirement, the individual should have some interest in the problems of the psychoses. A chemist, statistician, or psychologist should not be selected merely on the ground that he is a good man in his field but mainly because he is interested in applying his science to the problems of psychiatry. His best recommendation would be that he is proceeding from problems of mental disease to his science and not from his science to psychiatry.

He must be a research man. Technical proficiency is not enough. He must be research-minded and have had research training. It is not good administrative practice to say that we shall make a worker out of a good psychiatrist unless he has an inclination for such work. A man may be an excellent therapist or child guidance expert and be a dismal failure as a research worker. If his record shows that he has the proper inclination, he will work himself into the problems of the psychoses in a reasonable time. The true research man delights in any legitimate project. Care in the selection of workers in all fields of research is even more essential than on the regular staff. The standards for both should be high but different.

Having selected the proper individual, a carefully organized procedure should be put into effect to initiate him into the group. He should be made thoroughly acquainted with the hospital, its ideals and goal, its routine standard practice, and its departments. This is necessary that he may never lose sight of the fact that he is working in a mental hospital where the main responsibility is to treat and cure patients. It should also be brought home to him that he makes a negative or a positive contribution to this goal, both directly and indirectly—directly by his example, knowledge, and leadership in his field, and indirectly by the knowledge he may pass on through his research activities. Having become saturated with the hospital atmosphere, he proceeds to go through an integrating process by thoroughly familiarizing himself with every research department.

LEADERSHIP

Assuming that the proper personnel has been selected, morale will depend upon leadership. Research workers are subject to the same psychological techniques that other workers are. For successful creative work it is necessary that all workers have confidence in the plan. Before they can have such confidence they must know what the scheme is. And if the leader has no plan, they are soon aware of it. It would be helpful to have the general plan of the research charted in order to present it visually to the new worker. And this confidence must be manifested in the leader, otherwise the workers cannot have it. The latter must be convinced that the leader takes it seriously. He must create the impression that he is acquainted with all the activities and understands the complications and difficulties. This impression can only be created if he really does understand. Workers must also feel that the leader takes an interest not only in their work but in their personal selves. They must be convinced that he is working towards a definite goal and that they know the path which leads there.

Much of this leadership must, of necessity, fall upon the research director. But the administrator cannot completely escape from his responsibilities in this field. His interest, understanding, and sympathy are essential in any undertaking of this kind. Practically he can show this spirit by occasionally visiting a research department and discussing the problems, difficulties, and achievements with the workers. This cannot be done with the attitude of "What have you discovered today?" It must governed by a genuine enthusiasm for the work that is being done. This is coöperative research. It is likewise a participative democracy.

I am somewhat disturbed by the feeling that administrators who read this chapter may become alarmed by the complicated technique of organization which is outlined and decide that the results will not be worth the labor involved. Yet I cannot bring myself to paint a rosy picture which I know is not true. A research organization brings many heartaches, sleepless nights, and brain-storms to the administrator. It compels him to completely reorganize his thinking and particularly to broaden his conception of what constitutes that no-man's land through which normality passes into abnormality. Research men are not always practical in their thinking or even in their behavior, they unquestionably bump one out of ruts and not always in a kindly way, and they frequently have the conventionally trained executive gasping for breath. But in spite of these difficulties, the feeling that progress is being made towards a goal, that no matter how dark the present may be there is always the hope of turning the corner and finding a ray of light, the patient plodding with an occasional period of excitement when a new fact has been found, and the realization that one is making an effort to contribute to the health of our people more than compensate for the irritations, the risks, and the dangers that are present when research is a major interest of the hospital. This is the romance of research and it is worth all it costs in trouble and anxiety.

Chapter 12

CLINIC ORGANIZATION

This is the day of preventive medicine. Man is no longer content to cure the disease that makes him uncomfortable and unhappy, but he is definitely thinking in terms of how to prevent it. He is trying to anticipate illness. Psychiatry shows trends leading in the same direction. The entire mental hygiene scheme, with its accentuation of prophylaxis and prevention, is in line with the principles of modern preventive medicine. Prophylactic health measures have been successful only in proportion to the interest and coöperation that have been aroused in the general community. One of the outstanding examples of this is tuberculosis. There was a time when that disease stigmatized the patient exactly as mental disease does today. But through popular educational propaganda, carried on skillfully, constantly, and through a coördinated plan, the attention of the people was focussed on the preventive aspects of the disease and a mass movement initiated which is only now beginning to reflect itself in the incidence of the malady. Smallpox vaccination passed through similar experiences. The opposition to the procedure gradually lessened through the influence of popular education, and when the resistance was exemplified by only a minority of the group, the disease began to disappear and today is a negligible factor in public health.

But there is an important difference between these diseases and mental hygiene. The cause of tuberculosis was definitely known. That vaccination prevented smallpox had actually been established. In other words, scientific facts formed the basis of popular education and when the methods recommended were tried, results were achieved.

Mental hygienists have been preaching the doctrine of prevention in psychiatry for twenty-five years. Unfortunately much of the education was ill-advised and not supported by actual knowledge. A demand for preventive measures was created that far exceeded the psychiatric facilities and set up hopes which could not be realized. Research had lagged behind, the propagandist sold his product faster than it could be manufactured, and the result was loss of reputation for psychiatry. History shows that this is usually the case when a new movement is born. Enthusiasts make unfounded claims and the public, reacting to the emotional oratory of these individuals, rushes to absorb the panacea that will dissipate all personality difficulties and mental quirks. The inevitable result is disillusionment, followed by the reaction of lack of confidence and respect.

In spite of this there is still a demand on the part of the public for psychiatric clinics. That this is true is evidenced by the rapid development during the past decade of child and adult clinics. There is a definite swing away from the extravagant claims of early exponents of mental hygiene towards a recognition of the limitations of preventive psychiatry. While no specific preventive measures have been discovered, enough sound knowledge has accumulated to show that a continuance and extension of the clinic program is a logical procedure.

With this more reasonable attitude and the obvious need for the enlargement of clinic facilities, the State hospital comes into the picture. It must assume a prominent rôle and a position of leadership. Most of the extramural organizations that have come into existence since the mental hygiene crusade began have been fostered by private or semi-private agencies. Some have been unable to stem the engulfing tide of economic depression and because of lack of financial support have closed their doors. Others have survived but are not able to enlarge their scope of activity or extend their sphere of usefulness. These experimental clinics have served the useful purpose of doing the pioneer work, but it would seem that the time has arrived for a mass attack on the problems of preventive psychiatry. In this we must turn to the State hospital, because government is the only agency that is sufficiently powerful to bring into play a mass movement which will make a real impression on the incidence of mental disease and delinquency. The hospital systems that have been set up by every State in the union can be extended and utilized for community psychiatry, without creating more expensive machinery to add to the already crushing burden of taxation.

The majority of clinics now in operation are located in the large centers of population. The rural districts do not have this service, except in isolated instances. Yet the number of people served by the metropolitan clinics is so small compared with the actual needs of the total population that they can only accomplish a fraction of the good that would be possible if the more remote districts could be reached. There must be an equal distribution of clinic service between the urban and rural population.

The hospital has a proprietary interest in the problem of the pre-psychotic and delinquent child. The child guidance patient of today becomes the mental case of tomorrow. The patients who will be received by the institution ten, fifteen, twenty years from today are in our public schools and many of them are even now showing behavior abnormalities that stamp them as potential deviates. It seems clear that the State hospital has a grave responsibility in this field of prevention and must prepare to assume that duty as quickly as personnel can be secured and trained to do the work.

The State of Pennsylvania inaugurated a system of state hospital clinics in 1934 that was designed to reach every part of the Commonwealth. It was one of the most comprehensive and far-reaching plans that has been tried. Briefly the arrangement called for the organization of a therapeutic clinic unit in each hospital district, which was to serve the population of the area as a clinic for child guidance, for adults suffering from mental disease or neurological conditions, and for the examination of furloughed patients from the hospital. Each class is seen on a different day but the main emphasis is placed on child guidance. The plan as outlined carried out the principle of community participation which I believe to be essential to the success of any state-wide clinic project.

The stress laid upon work with children is entirely justifiable when one considers that prevention is most hopeful in childhood. It is the golden age for mental hygiene. For a state hospital program which has prevention as a goal, the child guidance clinic will be the important phase of preventive psychiatry. The organization of such a clinic by a mental hospital offers many difficulties that will tax the ingenuity of the administrator to overcome. It is hard for schools, social workers, and churches to grasp the fact that the hospital can have any interest beyond that of keeping patients locked up. Because of this attitude, attempts to organize a child study clinic may meet with suspicion and lack of understanding. If the administrator does not have the soul of a pioneer which enables him to persistently keep on in the face of many discouragements, his mental hygiene clinic will die before it is really born. His efforts will be facilitated if the hospital has carried on community educational propaganda as a part of its general service policy.

One of the early Child Guidance Clinics in this country fostered by a state hospital is the Worcester Child Guidance Clinic. This organization had a turbulent career until the past five years, when it began to emerge as a definite asset to the community. But during the formative period there were many times when it seemed to be moribund. It is out of this practical experience that the principles and policies discussed in this chapter have developed. The pitfalls are numerous and many of them dangerous to the success of the project. The constant interplay of community life creates hazards to the clinic that are difficult for the administrator to appreciate unless he has actually been through the experience. The ramifications of human lives into the social fabric are tortuous and deeply buried, and a community clinic cannot stand in the same detached position that the hospital can occupy. It is too much a part of the community. But in spite of mistakes and errors in judgment, the organization has survived the vicissitudes of time and made its place in society.

ORGANIZATION

The most outstanding fact that has come out of this experiment in mental hygiene is that citizens of the community play a very important part in the success of the clinic. I emphasize and re-emphasize this point to the extent of boredom, because I believe that few child psychiatrists actually appreciate the importance of it. I say without qualification that there can be no effective psychiatric treatment of children without community loyalty. Such a relationship does not generate spontaneously but only through organized effort. The announcement that the hospital intends to organize a children's clinic does not, as a rule, provoke much enthusiasm. People do not understand what such an organization stands for, and its association with a mental hospital brings out the fear and horror of mental disease that is prevalent. The connection between psychiatry and the behavior of children is not always clearly understood. Real opposition may develop among medical men who are quick to look at any extension of clinic facilities with a jaundiced eye. They are on guard to prevent state medicine, and while the hospital system is regarded with toleration, the profession is quick to resent any invasion of that system into community life. The tendency of administrators has been to take the establishment of a children's clinic rather lightly, at least as far as the relationship to the community is concerned. This attitude is a mistake that may prove to be costly in the end. Unless one appreciates the fact that a considerable amount of preparatory educational work must be carried out before actual treatment of patients begins, there may be no clients when the clinic opens. As an instance of this lack of understanding, a mental hospital executive decided to open a clinic in a certain town in his district. Having made arrangements to use the outpatient department of the general hospital as headquarters, he called one of the junior staff men and instructed him to open the clinic. One reason for the selection was the fact that the particular individual could best be spared from the hospital. The young man appreciated his own lack of experience and understanding. But like a good soldier, he obeyed the chief. The clinic, if it could be dignified by that name, staggered along for a brief period and then quietly folded up. The reaction of the community towards this abortive attempt prevented child guidance from being established for a long period of time. From six months to a year is not too long to spend in plowing the ground and preparing it for the seed. This preparation must be a period of organization and education. The average man has little understanding of this kind of work with children. He is apt to think that the clinic is interested only in feebleminded or psychotic individuals. And it is not easy to explain clearly just what the psychiatrist does for the child.

The preliminary measures should be carried on by the man who is to direct the clinic. It is important that he be identified as a part of the city or town in which the organization is working. Outsiders do not fit well with the town people, who frequently resent anyone coming into their city and telling them facts which they know but will not admit. The director must have a personality which enables him to ingratiate himself into the local situation. He must be accepted, and this will be his own personal responsibility. He will make his own position in the community and no amount of influence on the part of the administrator will accomplish the result for him.

A Child Guidance Clinic, of all social agencies, should not be attached to any organization that would subject it to local political pressure. The only exception to this would be a clinic that is in the very small community where, from motives of economy, it may be a part of the school system. It must be free from all entangling alliances and particularly those which make it dependent upon any local group. The clinic must be free to serve all without fear or favor. And in this respect the State hospital is in a strategic position. Being a state-controlled organization, it can keep aloof from local difficulties.

It is essential that the Child Guidance Clinic have as many influential people as possible supporting it, and every method of publicity must be used to get this interest. If the hospital is located in or near the town in which the clinic is to be, public meetings at the institution are an excellent way to break down the barrier between community and hospital, and in time citizens will appreciate and understand the desire of the administor to carry out a program of prevention.

It is of advantage to have a regularly organized group behind a clinic movement, such as a Women's Club or Junior League. But here the administrator will step carefully because such support may become embarrassing. Community jealousies and antagonisms are strong, and to get a clinic involved in one of these feuds will interfere very materially with its success and prestige. The logical society to sponsor such a movement is a State or local Mental Hygiene Association. This should be in line with the work of such a group, and the experience of the director in public propaganda would be of great assistance in these preliminary measures. Or it may be preferable to organize a Child Guidance Association, the sole object of which would be to act as the supporting body. The Worcester Clinic created such a group, which has grown into a very efficient and strong organization. It has no divided purpose and the energies are not scattered. Membership is made up of representatives of social agencies, teachers, physicians, clergymen of every faith, lawyers, judges, business men, and parents. It is a cross-section of the community. As many influential citizens as possible must be interested and induced to accept membership. The group will eventually have a financial responsibility in the clinic. While this question cannot be emphasized in the early stages of development, it must come sooner or later because the interest of the group will be in direct proportion to the financial responsibility. Our experience is that the sooner the sponsoring organization accepts this fact, the earlier the clinic will enjoy community prestige. A fair division of expense between state and town is for the latter to furnish proper quarters, clerical assistance, and maintenance costs, while the former supplies professional personnel. If the town or city has a community chest organization, steps should be taken to apply for membership and secure financial assistance in this way. Naturally the methods used by the hospital administrator will vary with local conditions, but this point of community interest must be kept in mind if the maximum amount of result is to be achieved.

CLINIC ORGANIZATION

Location. The principal question which confronts the administrator is whether the clinic shall be located at the hospital. There are many reasons why this is not the best policy, even though the institution has the respect and confidence of the community. Even housing it in a detached building on the institution grounds is a procedure of questionable wisdom. The Child Guidance Clinic will be stronger and enjoy a better reputation if its close connection with the state hospital is not stressed. The suggestion conveyed to parents through a physical association of clinic and hospital may provoke a very violent reaction. In spite of considerable progress towards a more healthy attitude in regard to mental disease, the old ideas of disgrace and stigma die hard. The time may, and it is to be hoped, will come when the mental hospital may openly proclaim its interest in these mental hygiene matters. But that time has not yet arrived, and until it is here, the prejudices of the people must be taken into consideration.

It is not good technique in child guidance work to mix children with adults and particularly psychotics. The experience of those whose own children have grown up in the atmosphere of a mental hospital shows that such surroundings do not constitute the best environment. The mere fact that a child must be brought to the hospital may seriously affect the rapport of the clinic with both parents and child. A Child Guidance Clinic in such a location will not be able to do its best work.

When housed on the hospital grounds, identification with the community is lost. It is a part of the institution, and as such, the interest in the work rapidly diminishes. The hospital is frequently located in such relation to the town that transportation would be a serious difficulty. Any location is preferable to the hospital itself, and yet if it comes to a choice between such a plan and no clinic, it would be better to have the clinic. The best contact the hospital can have is through such an organization, and the administrator can find no better method of increasing the influence of his institution than by a Child Guidance Clinic.

General Hospital

While no general statement can be made except that local conditions will govern location, our experience indicates that the general hospital is not an ideal place to house a juvenile psychiatric clinic. The medical profession must go a long way before it can fully understand and sympathize with the work of those who are interested in the mental and emotional life of children. The scientific atmosphere which permeates the hospital does not lend itself to such studies. In those institutions where psychiatric departments have been organized the situation is different, and it is to be hoped that the number of such progressive hospitals will rapidly increase. With the emphasis that is being placed upon the somatopsychic relationship in all branches of medicine, I believe that very soon we shall see the child guidance clinic where it should be—a part of the pediatric department of the general hospital. But at present in most communities the clinic, if accepted at all in the general hospital, is on sufferance. Because of crowded conditions, adequate office space is rarely available, and the clinic that has to work in cramped space will not be able to render the best type of service. The frenzied haste and bustling activity that is characteristic of the busy general hospital is not an atmosphere in which children can be treated psychiatrically. To establish a good rapport with them, the psychiatrist must do his work in a reasonably calm and leisurely atmosphere. Children cannot be hurried or pushed about.

If the general hospital organization has the proper understanding of the clinic and the desire to make it a part of the institution, there are advantages in such a location. The facilities can be used freely and with a minimum of inconvenience to both clinic and patients. It gives the director an opportunity to render a consultation service to the general profession and through this to develop a better relationship. But while these are obvious benefits, they can only be realized under special conditions which unfortunately prevail in all too few communities.

SOCIAL AGENCY BUILDING

In many communities a number of social agencies are housed in a single building, and the clinic which has quarters in such a place is in an advantageous position. In our present stage of psychiatric development, it is preferable to the general hospital. The clinic is housed in an atmosphere of understanding and the relationship engendered by close contact with many agencies is apt to be a healthy and profitable one. The community identification becomes stronger and there is an excellent opportunity for the psychiatric education of general social workers through the clinic service. The disadvantage of such an arrangement is the danger of becoming identified with one agency or group of agencies, with the accompanying risk of the services of the clinic being monopolized by a few. This may involve the organization in undesirable local situations and will certainly limit the sphere of usefulness. Such complications should be avoided by every Child Guidance Clinic.

Office Building

There are many advocates of this plan and it undoubtedly has merits. Some of the most successful guidance clinics have been housed in office buildings. The patients come to the clinic as they would go to any physician's office and there is no feeling of stigma. Psychologically it is sound. If the group can be located in a so-called medical building, the opportunity for better rapport with the profession is decidedly improved and there will be less isolation. The main disadvantage is the noise and confusion of the city streets. Children are distractible and the hum of traffic and the sounds of life which strain through the stoutest walls are apt to be a disturbing factor in the physician-child relationship.

Private Residence

Most directors of Child Guidance Clinics agree that this is the ideal location. If the house is on a quiet side street, sufficiently near the business section to be convenient but far enough away to escape the bustle and confusion, the setting is best for the child. It should be near a car or bus line and have parking facilities. The Worcester Child Guidance Clinic occupies a fourteen-room dwelling on a quiet, tree-lined street and is adjacent to a small general hospital. The house is owned by the Worcester Child Guidance Association, an incorporated body, and was purchased with money subscribed by citizens of Worcester. This is the community financial responsibility. The affairs of the association are managed by an executive committee of five. The charter of the corporation provides that the superintendent of the State hospital, the director of the clinic, and the chief psychologist of the clinic must be members of this committee.

To illustrate this state-community relationship, the Worcester Child Guidance Clinic is offered as a unique plan of organization which has worked successfully for a number of years. The clinic is financed from three sources:

1. Commonwealth of Massachusetts
2. Worcester State Hospital
3. Community Chest of the City of Worcester

The bulk of the finances comes from the State through a special appropriation from the legislature. This money is given to the Department of Mental Diseases for the specific purpose of supporting the clinic. It is disbursed through the hospital. The contribution of the institution is mainly in the maintenance of clinic personnel. The director and other members of the staff live on the hospital grounds. This is an economical procedure. The Community Chest of the city supports the house in which the clinic is lodged and supplies clerical assistance, office supplies, telephone and travel expense. The proportion of each is approximately 75 per cent for the State and 25 per cent for the city. This is an equitable distribution of the financial burden.

It is an interesting fact that most of the money paid for this house was raised through the efforts of the Women's Auxiliary of the Worcester State Hospital, an organization composed of the wives of the professional and lay staff of the institution. The financial support of the citizens gives the community an interest in the work being carried on. The clinic is used by juvenile courts, social agencies, physicians, and parents, and in the minds of these people it is a local enterprise. But because of the support of the State it has some independence and can keep out of local situations that might prove embarrassing. In this setting and with the personalities involved, the arrangement has proven to be very satisfactory. Furthermore the plan gives financial security to the staff. The director does not have to spend his time raising money. He need not concern himself about appropriations because these matters are handled by the superintendent of the hospital. Modifications of the plan to meet different conditions would be necessary, but it does carry out the principle that I believe is essential—that both city and state must share the burden. A hospital clinic without the assistance of the citizens will never be able to enlist the interest of the public as will one that is organized in this fashion.

Rural Organization

I am not unmindful of the fact that a plan which is successful in a city of 200,000 may not meet the needs of towns with a population of 2,000, and hospitals located where communities are small and far apart will have to work out modifications which will meet their necessities. Where there are no cities large enough to justify the existence of a permanent, full-time organization, the traveling clinic is the alternative. To have a group from the mental hospital go into a small town one day a week or month, examine certain children who are referred by teachers or parents, make a diagnosis, recommend treatment, and then leave until the next clinic day is, in my opinion, not an organization that will give the maximum amount of service. There must be some local relationship that brings the work closer to the people. In this situation the state hospital can make a combination of hospital and community in one of two ways. One is to attach the clinic to the public school system and organize a nucleus of local school attachés who will carry on work with simple problems, with the hospital personnel acting in an advisory capacity. The latter group can visit the community several days each month for conference and to see special cases in which the problems are unusually difficult and involved. In the school system the school physician, visiting teacher, and school nurse constitute the permanent clinic, while the hospital supplies psychiatrist, social worker, and psychologist. With this community coöperation, one institution unit can efficiently manage Child Guidance Clinics in from ten to twelve small towns.

The other plan that might be possible, under certain conditions, is to utilize the services of physicians in practice who have had mental hospital experience. Many physicians who have served on the staff are capable of organizing and directing such a clinic. To the administrator who sees the need of such an extension of the hospital service, ways and means will be found and the entire district from which the hospital receives patients will be organized into a mass approach to the problem of mental disease and delinquency.

Always must we emphasize to the citizens that this is not a responsiblity to be shoved off onto the State but one which they should prepare themselves eventually to carry on independently and with a minimum amount of assistance from the hospital. The same careful and thorough preparatory educational work that is so essential in the metropolitan area must be done in the small town.

CLINIC POLICIES

Before a clinic is organized, certain policies should be carefully considered and a decision made by the advisory committee as to the order of importance of these functions and the relative proportion of time that should be given to each. It is true that the actual determination of this important matter must be made by the administrator, because he has the experience and expert knowledge. As a matter of education, the committee should be asked to assist in the policy-making deliberations. The consideration of this vital matter will hinge on four points:

1. Therapy
2. Teaching
3. Research
4. Public Education

The relative importance of these will change from time to time as the prestige of the clinic increases. At the outset a larger proportion of time must be given to public education than is necessary after the period of organization has passed. In fact much of the director's time and energy must be expended in this field during the early stage of development.

Therapy. The most momentous decision the committee must make is the policy to be followed regarding the function of the clinic. Is it to be a diagnostic organization or will therapy be the real purpose? I suppose no Child Guidance Clinic director would admit that his work was largely diagnosis, but practically that is what it will be unless there is a very definite policy of regulating intake. The case-load of the psychiatrist must be held down to a point where he can actually devote sufficient time to each child to accomplish something therapeutically. I doubt if any psychiatrist can, in addition to his administrative duties, see more than three children each day and give much to each. We have found in the Worcester Clinic that a staff consisting of director, assistant psychiatrist, two psychologists, and four social workers can treat only 250 new cases a year. More than this means that proper attention cannot be given to each child. A Guidance Clinic requires leisure and calm if the children are to be treated and not merely diagnosed. Modern efficiency methods have no place in such an organization, at least in the actual treatment of the child and his problems.

Therefore the group which is working out the clinic policies must be prepared to consider frankly the proper course to follow. The pressure to take children for study will be tremendous if the proper personnel is in charge. Of course if the director and his assistants are not well trained and do not make good community contacts, the question need give no concern because the clinic will not be patronized by those who need it. The selection of a director is, to some extent, governed by the policy of functioning decided upon. I cannot see why any clinic should be other than one where therapy is the prime consideration. But unless a very clear and unequivocal policy is decided upon and adhered to in spite of all pressure, it is bound to become a center for diagnosis rather than treatment.

Teaching. What should the attitude be towards the utilization of the organization for educational purposes? And if personnel is to be trained, how much time should be devoted to this aspect of the work? These are questions that the administrator and his committee must settle. Obviously trained people are needed in Child Guidance Clinics, and as these increase in number, more people will be required. It would seem that every clinic should make some contribution by participating in an educational program. But to give an undue prominence to this phase of the work to the detriment of therapeutic considerations is unwise and will eventually prove disastrous.

Research. In the field of research every clinic has a responsibility. If the Child Guidance movement is to continue and actually achieve results by decreasing the incidence of mental disease and delinquency, we must be willing to check progress regularly. To go on accumulating data year after year without assimilating and digesting them is absurd. To go on studying children without making some attempt to find out what has happened to them after a lapse of five, ten, or fifteen years is not a scientific attitude. Child Guidance techniques are still crude, our basis of factual knowledge is inadequate, and we are still in the dark about much that governs the behavior of children. Every clinic has some responsibility in this field. It cannot be over-emphasized but should be given its proper value.

Public Education. Public education must occupy a large proportion of the work of the newly organized clinic. As the organization is accepted and its work more generally understood, the need for undue emphasis on this aspect gradually diminishes. It never quite disappears, and clinic staffs must always devote some time to community education. It should be pointed out, however, that the wrong kind of educational propaganda may do more harm than good. We should never promise more than can be delivered. Information must be founded on facts and not upon wish fulfilment. Conservative, well-founded statements command respect; wildly exaggerated and absurd claims only provoke ridicule and loss of respect for the enterprise.

PERSONNEL

A. *Director.* The mental hospital Child Guidance Clinic will reflect the director. He is the pivot about which the entire project revolves. No mental hospital administrator has the time to be the head of the clinic organization and if he had, it is questionable whether his experience and training would qualify him for the position. He can counsel and advise but in the end he and his advisory group must select as director the man who has the best qualifications that can be secured for the money available, give him the authority and responsibility to proceed, and pray that a wise choice has been made. The directorship of either an adult or child clinic is a full-time position. A successful clinic will not remain so long if it is the secondary responsibility of anyone. The time and energy necessary for the maintenance of community relationships, the treatment of individual patients, and the educational and research work to be done demand all of the director's time. The practice of delegating a staff member to do the work of a children's clinic is, in my opinion, unwise. No man is capable of making the mental and emotional transition from the problems of the adult psychotic to those of a child within the space of a few hours. The human mind is incapable of such rapid adjustment over such a wide area. The directorship is a full-time position for a trained man, capable of dealing with children. Child guidance is a specialty of psychiatry and as such calls for individuals who are fitted for the work by education, training, and personality.

What should these qualifications be?

1. I believe that the director should be a physician, a graduate of a class A medical school, and with a two-year general internship in an approved general hospital. In spite of the tendency of some psychiatrists to put the major emphasis in children's problems upon psychogenetic and environmental factors, the physical aspect cannot quite be eliminated. Therefore a physician with a mind always alert to the possibility of disease is a decided asset. Sex is of no importance except in special situations.

2. He should have at least two years' experience on the staff of a progressive mental hospital with an active admission rate. Adult psychiatry is indispensable to the clinic worker. Inasmuch as a considerable percentage of the work is carried on with parents, an understanding of the adult is essential.

3. He should have spent a minimum of one year, and preferably two years, in a Child Guidance Clinic under a director who is actually capable of training personnel. During this time he should have experience in every phase of the work—administration, public relations, therapy, pedagogy, and research.

4. He must have a personality that is suited to work with children. While he has to be objective, there must always be a certain emotional attitude towards his patients that impels them to accept him.

5. He must have some organizing and administrative ability. The clinic connection with the hospital makes it imperative that certain rules and regulations be followed, especially in financial matters. His organizing ability is shown by his

relationships with agencies. He must be able to keep on friendly terms with all and at the same time not relax in the fundamental principles that have been laid down.

6. He must have the ability to speak convincingly and with sincerity before groups. He should have a common-sense attitude towards psychiatry and particularly Child Guidance. He should have some teaching competency and be interested in research to the point where he can stimulate others to have a critical feeling about their own work.

7. He must be able to see in the relationship with the State hospital an opportunity for advancing and extending the scope of Child Guidance. He should be able to appreciate and utilize the resources of the institution. A holier-than-thou attitude is not justified and renders an individual useless in this kind of set-up.

8. And finally he must have sufficient leadership qualities to weld his group together into a harmonious team. In no phase of psychiatry is the coöperative approach so important as in the Child Guidance Clinic.

B. *Chief Social Worker*. The relationship between the director and chief social worker is an intimate one. She concerns herself with problems of family adjustment, while the psychiatrist works with the patient. They are the leading members of the clinic team. Her background and experience must be carefully considered by director, administrator, and committee.

1. She should be a graduate of a recognized school of social work and have had at least one year's experience in family case work.

2. Graduation from a psychiatric social service school is essential.

3. She should have at least one year on the social service staff of a mental hospital.

4. She should have at least two years' experience as a salaried social worker on the staff of a recognized Child Guidance Clinic.

5. She must have those personality traits that enable her to pull her share of the load. The responsibility for the leadership of social workers is hers and much of the relationship with community agencies will be of her making.

6. The chief social worker must be capable of addressing

public groups, have some pedagogical ability, and have a considerable amount of executive efficiency.

C. *Chief Psychologist.* This is the one position in the clinic that need not be full-time until the load increases to the point where his services are constantly in demand. But he must be more than a psychometrist. He is an indispensable member of the team and his qualifications should be such that he is capable of occupying a chief rôle in the clinic conferences. He must be able to see in his work more than the mere finding of a mental age.

1. He must have an M.A. degree in psychology from a school in which the psychological department is emphasized.
2. He should have had at least two years' training in abnormal psychology.
3. He should have had at least one year in work with children under an experienced psychologist, preferably in a Child Guidance Clinic.
4. He must have the type of personality that will enable him to work with a group.

These are the individuals upon whom the success of the clinic will depend. Like every other department of the hospital, the results of Child Guidance will reflect the ability of the staff and will be no better or no worse than the members make it. And the ability of that staff will be no better than the administrator will permit it to be.

ADMINISTRATION OF CLINIC—CLASSIFICATION OF CASES

Cases coming to a Child Guidance Clinic for treatment and study do not lend themselves to a definite classification. When arranged in groups one always finds an overlapping from one into another. No case is a pure culture of any one problem. But there is always an outstanding part of the real problem, if it can be found, which makes it possible to effect a rough arrangement of cases which is classification. The chief advantages of doing this are: first, some evaluation may be made of the type of cases that are best and most usefully treated in the clinic; second, a general idea may be gained of the type of case from which society will derive the most help, providing a successful result is obtained in any considerable per cent of the cases; and third, some general idea may be gained of where the amount of clinical effort that may be brought to bear on the total case load may be best expended. The following classification is used in the Worcester clinic:

I. *Physical Diseases and Abnormalities*
   (Where the behavior or personality problems are primarily on an organic basis)

II. *The Convulsive Disorders*
   A. Probably Psychogenic
   B. Organic or Probably Organic

III. *Intellectual Handicaps*
   A. Special Problems of Highly Superior Child
   B. " " " Dull Child
   C. Problems of Feebleminded
   D. Special Disabilities

IV. *Emotional Traumata*
   (Such as suddenly broken bones, sudden or tragic death of relatives or comrades, attempts on child's life, sexual assaults, etc.)

V. *Environmental*
   A. Material
      (Poverty, bad neighborhoods, desertion of child, etc.)
   B. Attitudes of Parents
      1. Over-protection
      2. Rejection and Antagonisms
      3. Misunderstandings
   C. Attitudes of Others

VI. *Mental Conflicts*
   A. Conscious Conflicts
      (Major part of emotional problem recognized by child)
   B. Unconscious or suppressed conflicts
      (Where major part is not recognized)

VII. *Neurotics*
   A. Anxiety States
   B. Transference Neuroses
   C. Obsessional Compulsive

VIII. *Psychopathic Personalities*
   A. Pre-Psychotic
   B. Psychotic

SOURCE OF REFERRALS

A. *Agencies*
   1. Social (including non-medical institutions)
   2. Medical and Health

B. *Schools*
   1. Public
   2. Private
   3. Parochial

C. *Courts*
   1. Juvenile
   2. Adult

D. *Private Physicians*

E. *Parents, Relatives, Self*

PITFALLS

Unwarranted dogmatism on the part of the clinic staff is ruinous. There is no justification for such an attitude and it will cause antagonism towards the clinic. The administrator who is unwilling to accept modern, dynamic psychiatry must keep his prejudices in the background. If he cannot do this it would be better not to embark on the clinic project. The director who is an ardent disciple of Freud or one of his allied schools of thought must temper his enthusiasm if he is not to create dissatisfaction. If there is anyone in psychiatry who should humbly admit his limitations in the face of conduct problems, it is the man or woman who works with children. The book of child psychology and behavior still has many pages that are written in a language we cannot read. And a cocksure belief that any one explanation of child behavior is correct is not the feeling that leads eventually to scientific truth. We must avoid, like the plague, an opinionated insistence that the last word has been spoken and keep an open mind towards all methods of approach.

The parent is an important factor in any situation where

children's problems are involved. Without the coöperation of these individuals, the psychiatrist can do little for the child. They cannot be eliminated from the situation. There are so many psychological circumstances working in these parents that the psychiatrist cannot afford to be too radical in his attitude. The sense of guilt may be strong in either father or mother. Parents may have a vague idea that they are responsible in some way for the child's difficulties. The sense of shame enters into the situation. Hurt family pride is a powerful factor which operates too often. Resentment against life and what it has brought is another factor. These and many other feelings and emotions confuse the issue and draw red herrings across the trail of the real trouble. The psychiatrist who treats the child exclusively will probably not get very far in correcting the difficulty.

Child Guidance psychiatrists have created many difficulties for themselves by not taking into consideration the ideas of the community regarding sex topics. Radical advice along any line does not help the clinic, and birth control and sex subjects discussed in an unrestrained way will do much to injure both clinic and hospital in the eyes of the people. No one regrets more than the writer that free information cannot always be given on these matters, but the fact still remains that the administrator must bear the burden of criticism and the director who has no correct sense of diplomacy in these fields will do incalculable harm. We must force ourselves to go no faster than the public can follow, if we expect to retain our psychiatric leadership.

Clergymen of all faiths should be strong supporters of a children's clinic, and they will be if the director will make them allies. And yet many facts that have been learned about the behavior of children and adults are at variance with their training and it requires considerable time and energy to correct certain impressions. Conduct that is most dangerous from the standpoint of mental hygiene may be looked upon by the world as being meritorious. Special groups like clergymen, teachers, and others who are close to the lives of other human beings should be objects of special concern to the director in his educational efforts.

The medical profession needs a great deal of attention in

these mental hygiene matters. General physicians do not coöperate well with the Child Guidance Clinic. It is largely indifference and lack of understanding that prevents a close relationship. But there is no better way to gain the respect of the doctor in the community than to have a clinic director who knows his way about in the field of internal medicine. At least he must be sufficiently interested in this phase of his problem to utilize the medical resources of his own and other hospitals. The discouraging lack of interest in psychiatry shown by the profession is partly due to the medical school and is to some extent the fault of psychiatrists themselves. Until medical schools recognize that a proper understanding of the mental and emotional life of the individual is as important as a knowledge of his physiology and anatomy, it will not be possible to get the active interest of physicians. But this fact should not deter the director from making an attempt to get a better relationship with them. If he can gain their respect, he will have enlisted a group of powerful allies.

Both administrator and clinic staff will have black days of discouragement because of the lack of intelligent interest on the part of the community. Human nature is never so cruel and callous as when it turns a deaf ear to the problems of others, and this is always the case when our own difficulties are not pressing too heavily upon us. Psychiatric treatment of children is not spectacular. It performs no miracles. Usually the methods and techniques are so simple when explained to the layman that he sees nothing that anyone could not do. The mysterious always commands his respect. To correct this attitude is a Herculean and never-ending task in which both hospital and clinic have an equal responsibility. Both organizations must get results in the form of treatment of patients. They will have to give real service as the first and most important consideration. And in addition to this efficiency, both hospital and clinic will be forced to carry on persistently and constantly educational propaganda which reaches every part of the community they serve. This will be efficiently done only as the hospital administrator is convinced of the necessity of it. And after many years of these efforts, it may bear fruit in an increased public confidence in both organizations. Child

Guidance is not a field for the executive who is looking for immediate results.

There are certain dangers that beset the Child Guidance social worker. One of these, and perhaps the most important, is the attitude of the general social agencies towards psychiatric social work. There has grown up in the latter group an isolationist policy that will do a great deal of harm if it is permitted to continue. The attitude of superiority assumed by many psychiatric social workers towards the general worker is not the best way in which to render service. In my opinion the designation "psychiatric" is an unfortunate one. All social service would be improved if its representatives were trained psychiatrically, and psychiatric social service would be better if workers had more experience in general case work. Frequently the success or failure of the clinic is, to some extent, dependent upon how well its social workers meet this difficulty. All community social workers must be respected, and the best clinic worker is the one who shows by her understanding of general case work that she does respect the contributions of the general agency.

While the prejudice against the State hospital is still strong, the clinic social worker will be a powerful factor in intensifying or changing this public attitude. Her personal feeling about the institution will largely determine the emotions of those who come in contact with her. If she has a full and complete understanding of the aims and purposes of the hospital and sympathizes with such policies, she will have a powerful influence upon the thinking of others. But if she does not believe in the goal of the institution and is apologetic in her presentation of the work of the organization, she will be a positive menace as far as the hospital is concerned.

While this chapter largely concerns the Child Guidance Clinic organized by the mental hospital, it should be remembered that adult clinics are equally important in the mental hygiene program. The points discussed are applicable to this phase of outpatient activity. There are some modifications that are desirable. Location is not so important as it is with the children's clinic. I believe that the desirable place for the headquarters of a clinic for adults is the hospital, either mental or general. The dangers that were pointed out in the other connection do not hold true in this field. The necessity for the extension of the psychiatric approach to the general hospital patient is constantly becoming more apparent. When we speak of prevention it is important to realize that true prevention of some psychoses is in the study of physical disease. For instance, the prevention of general paresis is actually tied up with the public health question of syphilis. If this disease could be eliminated there would be no paresis. The arteriosclerotic and senile psychoses are intimately tied up with these physical conditions. If they could be prevented there would be no psychosis. The mental hospital psychiatrist would be a valuable asset to any general outpatient service in studying the reaction of the patient to his disease. An alliance with general medicine will be of the greatest importance in preventive psychiatry. The work being carried on in gastro-intestinal disorders is a case in point. That there is a relationship between certain gastro-intestinal diseases and the emotions no one can deny, but the exact influence cannot be determined without further clinical study and observation.

The community work in prevention will be an ever-increasing responsibility of the mental hospital in those states where the policy of placing the emphasis upon prevention and cure has been adopted. While the immediate results of such a program will only be an increase in the cost of operating the hospital, eventually such a program will contribute to a reduction in the number of first admissions to hospitals with a corresponding decrease in the financial burden. The sooner hospital administrators agree that this is a logical course to pursue and utilize their position of leadership to bring it about, the more rapidly will we bring that mass attack on mental disease which I believe is essential to making any impression upon its incidence.

Chapter 13

PUBLIC RELATIONSHIPS

If the mental hospital is to do good work it must have the sympathy and support of the community. The walls of ignorance, superstition, and suspicion will have to be torn down and a friendly relationship established. They will have to be demolished stone by stone. When this is accomplished, we shall let in a flood of the sunlight of public approval and the result will benefit both the institution and the community.

The supernatural attitude towards mental disease has not entirely disappeared. The medieval beliefs about mental aberration still exist to a greater extent than is commonly realized. Most of it is subconscious and therefore more dangerous and more difficult to eradicate. The only answer to this is public education, a long and never-ending process. The burden and responsibility of doing this is on the hospital. The public will not come to us.

Medical men have a repugnance to anything that smacks of advertising. Mental hospital administrators, being medical men, have often failed to grasp the importance of properly organized educational propaganda. One superintendent says,

> "We put all of our time, energy, and money into the efforts to give our patients good care. The best advertisement is a satisfied patient. Service will always advertise the hospital. It is foolishness to spend money telling the community what you are doing. Give the right kind of service and the public will learn all about the institution from the patient."

This is an attitude that is common to many hospital administrators. But a moment's reflection will show that it is not correct. In the first place the mental hospital will get advertising whether the administrator wants it or not. Usually it is the wrong kind. Frequently the administrator does not know of it. The term "satisfied patient" is an uncertain one. The patient may be satisfied that the hospital aided in his recovery, but he may also feel that the food was not good or that some particular nurse or physician did not treat him as he thinks he should have been treated. And these are the things he talks about.

Hospital publicity must be dignified, interpretative, and educational. It must constantly stress the fact that the institution is part of the community. The public must learn that hospital psychiatrists are not individuals who have failed to make a living in their profession and have had to crawl in under the beneficent protection of a State government, and that mental nurses are not uneducated, illiterate, and brutal individuals who show their sadistic tendencies by mistreating patients. We must teach society that mental hospitals are directed by honest, well-trained, scientific men who are trying to render service to the patient, and that mental nursing calls for training, character, personality, and enthusiasm for an ideal. A sense of proprietorship and community loyalty can only be built slowly and laboriously but it must be one of the goals of our educational program.

Hospitals that are handicapped by the interference of politics and politicians can best meet and correct this situation by a program of ethical publicity. The politician uses this weapon himself and well understands the power of it. It would be a bold man who would dare attack the institution in which the people had confidence. He would cease attempting to trade on the illnesses of human beings for his own personal aggrandizement if the hospital would set out systematically to educate the people as to its needs.

According to Ralph Welles Keeler,[87] "good will" does not come accidentally. It must be created. The process is long and continuous. It may be built by:

Letting the community know that the hospital has a real service to be given.

Convincing people that they need what it has to offer.

Making it easy to obtain.

Making people glad that they have what the institution has to offer.

The goal of such educational effort should be more than to add to the prestige of the hospital. The ultimate purpose should be mental health. No program of mental hygiene can ever hope to be successful which does not take into consideration the State hospitals. The mental hygienist cannot always be successful. There must be commitments, and the understanding psychiatrist knows when to utilize the resources of the institution.

The question is frequently asked, "What do you do to get a patient well besides locking him up?" "What medicine can be given to cure mental illnesses?" "Is surgery of any value?" An attempt to classify the actual therapeutic procedures of a mental hospital brings out some rather startling results. Just what does the institution do for the patient beyond segregating him from the community? General statements can be made regarding therapy. But to classify the therapeutic procedures and what they accomplish offers difficulties that few administrators realize until they have tried to do it. Any educational program should include the therapeutic program of the hospital. A full analysis of the resources of the mental hospital will give plenty of material for popular talks that are highly educational. The individual taxpayer is not so much interested in the amount of money that is being spent as he is in what he is getting for this money.

The hospital that thinks only in terms of the cure of patients is not fulfilling its function to the fullest extent. This is the day of preventive medicine. Psychiatry should be thinking in terms of prevention as well as cure. It should be a primary goal of every State hospital to formulate and carry out educational measures which are specifically directed towards the prevention of mental illness. But a real danger exists in too much enthusiasm for this particular phase of publicity. The education must not proceed any more rapidly than the actual results will justify. There has been in the past a strong tendency to "over-sell" mental hygiene. We have been prone to promise more than we can deliver. Conservative statements based upon actual knowledge and performance are proper. Startling information and exaggerated conclusions based upon insufficient data will do great harm to the whole movement.

Educational propaganda must be directed towards three sections of society:

A. The General Community
B. Special Groups
C. Relatives and Friends of Patients

The General Community. The world today is psychologically minded. It is receptive to information about mental hygiene presented in an understandable and attractive manner. The interplay in family relationships, the parent-child situation, the effect of our social life upon our personalities are all points of interest to the general community. The hospital that seeks to spread mental hygiene education among the people it serves will find a real demand for the service.

Lecture Bureau. The formation of a lecture bureau to supply speakers for clubs is an excellent way of rendering such service. In the organization of such a community division, the first step is to get together the staff members who are to do the speaking and formulate a program. Each speaker should have three or more popular lectures. The material of the talks should be edited, and it would be of distinct advantage to rehearse each speaker before the entire staff. The coördination of the material should be done by someone who has a feeling for this kind of propaganda. Public speaking should be a part of the training and duty of every staff member.

In preparing these talks certain important essentials must be kept in mind. Everyone cannot be an orator, but there is no man or woman who knows a subject and is enthusiastic about it who cannot talk convincingly.

Careful Preparation. The man who starts to speak with the explanation that he has not prepared a formal address need not make the statement. His audience knows this to be the case before he has uttered a dozen words.

Memorize the Talk. Unless one can speak readily and fluently from notes, it is preferable to memorize the address. Some people prefer to make a list of main topics on small cards. These serve as reminders in case there is a tendency to go astray. Those who cannot do this should memorize the speech.

Reading from Manuscript. If one cannot speak from notes and does not care to memorize what he is to say, one should read the address. Talks presented in this way are not well received, but it is better to read a paper than to stutter and stumble in an unintelligible manner.

Avoid Technical Terms. The audience does not have a psychiatric background. Never use a two-syllable word when a shorter one will express your meaning. Popular lectures are addressed to audiences made up of all grades of intellect. The dullest person in the audience should understand.

Make It Short. The speech should be long enough to cover the subject but short enough to be interesting. Time the speech carefully and stay within the time. One-half hour is as long as any scientific speaker can interest his audience. It is better for the audience to be disappointed that you have not spoken longer than to be glad that you are through.

Be Natural. Don't try to be funny unless you really are. Amateur speakers are seldom really humorous. But after all, the speaker is not an entertainer but a teacher. Leave the jokes to the radio comedians and be natural.

Enunciate clearly and speak loudly enough to be heard by those sitting in the last row. Too many medical men do what Irvin Cobb described as "holding a confidential conversation with the orchestra leader."

RADIO

Radio broadcasting has opened up great possibilities in psychiatric education. By means of it one may reach an audience of enormous proportions. Most radio stations welcome well-prepared talks dealing with mental health subjects. There are few hospitals that cannot secure the facilities of a local station for one or two series during the year. Even our own American Medical Association is broadcasting health information. Why should psychiatry lag behind?

In preparing radio material there is a special technique. The talks must be written exactly as they are to be given, and some stations require that they be submitted for censorship, in advance.

Each talk must be accurately timed. The average speaker

speaks at the rate of 150 words per minute. There are approximately 300 words of double-spaced typewritten material on an 8½" x 11" page. Therefore it will require two minutes to read one page of manuscript. In a fifteen-minute talk, two minutes should be allowed for the opening and closing announcements, therefore the actual speaking time is thirteen minutes. This means that the talk should cover six and one-half pages of double-spaced typewriting, which will be equivalent to about 2,000 words.

Clear enunciation is the secret of good radio speaking. Good diction is essential. Do not shout into the microphone but speak in a quiet, conversational tone. The same rules that were given in the case of public addresses follow in radio delivery. Many people get microphone fright, but after a trial or two one learns to get along without the stimulation of an audience.

MOVING PICTURES

The production of a moving picture film depicting the therapeutic activities which are utilized in the recovery of the patient is an effective method of education. Nothing should go into this film that cannot be related directly to the treatment of patients. Advertising the production of vegetables or the raising of cattle puts the hospital in the wrong light before the public. When the people of the community begin to talk about the wonderful farm or cattle the institution has, they overlook the fact that it is a curative organization.

Visual education is more efficient than verbal for the majority of people. Learning is facilitated by pictures, and the impressions made by a well-produced film will be deeper and more lasting than by any other means of public education.

The film cannot be just a series of unrelated pictures showing scenes about the institution but must be a well thought out production, using all the dramatic values possible, in order to get the idea across. Most of the hospital pictures I have seen do not meet this requirement. Showmanship is essential if such a film is to tell the actual story of what the hospital stands for. Most medical men shrink from this idea of dramatizing their institution. They insist that the story tell the bare truth without any drama. This is absurd. To tell such a story needs certain exaggerations and emphasis that can only be worked out by someone who has a sense of the dramatic.

The production of a picture which has dramatic value and presents a real story offers many difficulties for the amateur. The entire picture must be carefully considered and a complete scenario written before a scene is taken. The technical work requires a great deal of study and experimentation. If funds permit, a professional camera man with portable lighting units would give better results, and yet one of the best hospital pictures I have seen was made by the clinical director. When the necessity for a picture arises, the way can always be found.

USE OF MARIONETTES

One hospital made use of this very clever idea as part of the publicity program. The entire entertainment was designed for children. A play was written by the director of the children's clinic. This play served to bring certain mental hygiene facts to children. The occupational therapy department then designed and made a portable stage. The department made the marionettes and four aides rehearsed under the direction of the physician who wrote the play until they were able to do a professional job in putting across his ideas. The entertainment was offered to schools and met with a cordial reception from both teachers and children. The hospital marionettes were very popular. The preparation of them was an excellent project for a group of patients, and the time consumed in showing them was not great.

NEWSPAPER PUBLICITY

The attitude that many administrators take toward newspapers is an unfortunate one. The newspaper can and will be the best friend the hospital has, but there must be complete understanding between them. Each must appreciate the viewpoint of the other if events are to be judged in proper perspective. Suspicion does not engender confidence. The hospital administrator who frankly and freely discusses with a representative of the press any unusual situation that develops can be assured that he will receive fair treatment. The man who flies into a rage and damns the newspapers, who will not tell the facts or even see a reporter, need not be surprised if his hospital is shown in a bad light. He has no one but himself to blame.

Newspapers as well as hospitals are rendering a service to the community. They should have the same consideration and assistance in carrying out that purpose that is given to others. Newspaper men are human and react to fair treatment. They will work with the institution or against it, depending upon how much effort has been made to secure coöperation. One hospital administrator, recognizing the need for this coöperation, organized and carried through a definite program of education for the newspapers. He attacked the problem along these lines:

Personal Contacts. To initiate the movement he personally called on the city editor of each of the papers in the city where the hospital was located and approached the editor with this statement, "I believe that the relations existing between the hospital and your newspaper have not been what they should be. I recognize the fact that the newspaper has responsibilities that are as important as my own, and from now on I intend to give you real coöperation. If something unpleasant happens, I expect to call the papers and give them the unvarnished truth. It will not be necessary to feel that we are trying to cover up anything. I shall rely on your good sense and humanity to give this kind of news the proper value. If you feel that the institution should be criticized, I shall not complain provided the comment is based on accurate data.

"In return I ask two things:

"That your men keep in close touch with the hospital and give me a reasonable amount of time to create a background of understanding for what they write.

"That you do not publish any story which has not come from the hospital without giving me a chance to explain the facts."

The result of this policy has been that the relationship between hospital and newspapers is so cordial that even unpleasant publicity does little harm. The superintendent has faithfully kept his word. When an accident or suicide occurs, the city editor of each newspaper is called by telephone and the facts given him. Certain restrictions on these stories are well understood. Reporters never ask to photograph or interview patients. They know it is against the rules of the game to write flamboyant, sensational articles about scientific subjects. The request "Do not quote me directly on this" is always respected. The superintendent talks openly and freely to every newspaper man, and never has his confidence been abused.

Not only does the head of the institution deal with newspaper men on this basis, but every member of his staff is thoroughly familiar with his policies and meets reporters with the same frankness. No one in the hospital has any fear of publicity. The institution does not have to be on the defensive, knowing that frankness and open dealing is the only fair way to handle the situation and that the truth must be told to newspapers at all times.

Press Releases. The professional executive labors under the handicap of not always knowing what news is. The most trivial detail may be a good news story from the standpoint of the newspaper. The safe way to handle the matter is to send out a press release for everything that is out of the ordinary routine. The editor then uses his own judgment as to whether it can be used. The following summary of the kind of material that constitutes news was prepared by a newspaper man:

1. *Addresses of Staff Members.* When any member of the staff gives a talk before a community group a press release should be sent to the newspapers. This includes a brief abstract of what he will say. The communication can go several days before the talk is given, but there must be a release date on it. By sending a picture, the newspaper will gradually get all of the staff members in the "morgue."

2. *Meetings.* Mental hospitals have many meetings of psychiatric societies or medical associations. In preparing publicity for these give the following:

a. The officers of the society, with pictures of each.
b. A "Who's Who," covering any important persons who are to be present.
c. Abstracts of speeches and pictures of speakers.
d. Full program of meeting.

3. *Visitors.* Every mental hospital is visited at times by superintendents, state officials, or people who would be of interest to newspapers. If you know the individual is coming, send a press release for a certain date. It is possible that an interview and picture by the newspaper photographer would be desired.

4. *New Staff Members.* When finally engaging a new member of the staff ask for a photograph, and send this with a detailed history of his educational qualifications and experience.

5. *Staff Members Leaving the Hospital.* Send pictures and details of service.

6. *Internes and Students.* A group of internes or students would make a good story. Have pictures and names of individuals, with schools.

7. *Social Events.*

a. *Patients' Entertainments*
   Christmas Program
   Other Holiday Events
   Plays or other entertainments given by community group.
   Plays or other entertainments given by hospital personnel.

b. *Employees' Entertainments*
   Farewell Parties
   Benefit Dances
   Nurses' Alumnae Receptions
   Graduation Ceremonies

8. *Annual Report.* Abstract the annual report, using such material as you would like to have the public know about. Call attention to the needs of the hospital, what it is trying to accomplish, and the work it is doing. Do not fail to get in the number of discharges. The public is under the impression that no patient leaves a mental hospital, and anything that will show the fallacy of that belief is of value.

9. *New Equipment.* Any piece of new medical equipment purchased is news. Have several pictures and a full description of the apparatus.

10. *Suicides.* This is unpleasant publicity but one cannot play the game and not take the bitter with the sweet. The

mental hospital has the responsibility of many patients, no one of whom can live in the community. It is surprising that there are not more occurrences of this kind.

11. *Serious Accidents.* Accidents happen in mental hospitals, and why try to conceal the fact? Why not let the public know some of the difficulties that come with the responsibility of caring for a large group of mental cases?

12. *Escapes.* Mental hospitals are not prisons. When a patient leaves without permission there is no need for any great apprehension unless he has a history of violence.

Syndicate Articles. The mental hospital can make arrangements with newspapers in its district to publish regular stories dealing with mental hygiene matters. These can be prepared for daily or weekly distribution. They should appear regularly and be carefully prepared and edited. The best length is from 300 to 500 words, and each article must be written in popular style. This is one of the best ways of educating the general public in mental hygiene matters.

Service Clubs. Special groups like the Rotary, Kiwanis, Lions, Exchange, and Quota clubs are composed of the best citizens in the community. Entertaining these clubs at a noonday luncheon at infrequent intervals brings good will to the hospital. These organizations are influential and can strengthen the prestige of the institution.

SOCIAL RELATIONSHIPS OF THE STAFF

This is a most valuable publicity medium. The isolation of the mental hospital has always included the professional staff. Medical men who spend their full time in institutions tend to settle down to a social life that is bounded by the four walls. They have no contacts or community life except among those with whom they work. They feel no social responsibility and their lives are narrow and restricted. This is a serious mistake, both for the individual and the hospital. People judge the efficiency and integrity of any organization by the contact they have with the people who are connected with it. When the community meets a group of high-grade professional men and women who represent the mental hospital socially, the prestige of the latter is increased immeasurably. Membership in luncheon clubs, fraternal organizations, and churches all lead to relationships which are valuable to the institution as well as the individual. Mental hospitals have many traditions to handicap them, and one of the most vicious is that which requires the professional staff to live on the grounds. There is no more reason for compelling staff members to be constantly on call than there is for the industrial plant to require that its personnel live in the factory.

Another tradition which tends to prevent the complete utilization of the social life of the professional staff for educational publicity is the attitude towards the wives of staff members. From time immemorial they have been looked upon as interlopers. In fact it is only in recent years that many hospitals would have married men on the staff. And even today, the wife of the assistant is looked upon as an individual to be repressed and kept out of sight rather than as a possible asset to the institution. It is true that the tactless woman may become a nuisance under the present system of "living in," but these matters can always be controlled without treating every married woman who lives on the grounds as if she were an undesirable.

Special Groups

There are many special groups in the community which should be the object of special educational projects. The following are representative of these:

- Medical Societies
- Social Agencies
- Clergymen
- Nursing Organizations
- Legal Associations
- Police Departments

Medical Societies

It should be a requirement that every medical officer must belong to his local society and attend meetings. An interest in the professional group is to some extent a criterion of his enthusiasm and attitude. Psychiatry should be built upon a foundation of general medicine. The medical profession needs education along psychiatric lines as much as does the general population. The educational opportunities which come from the attendance of the staff at medical meetings cannot be overemphasized. But it should be stressed that more than a mere passive attendance is indicated. There should be some attempt made to assist in the direction of the society. In other words, the hospital staff should be leaders and not followers.

READING PAPERS BEFORE MEDICAL GROUPS

As frequently as possible staff members should be on the programs of local and state societies. I subscribe heartily to the idea that a paper should not be written unless there is something of importance to say, but I believe that the hospital psychiatrist has something to say to the general medical profession. It is a mistake to read complicated papers on psychiatric subjects which deal with involved mental mechanisms. Papers that are best received by the profession are those that they can understand in terms of their own interests.

HOSPITAL MEETINGS

Most mental hospitals have adopted the custom of entertaining the local society at least once each year. This is a splendid opportunity for educating the doctor. A well thought out program designed for educational purposes will do much to cement the bond of understanding between hospital and community.

HOSPITAL EXHIBITS

The medical profession has a rather vague understanding of psychiatry and in many cases scant respect for the men who practice it. There is no better way to show them what a hospital is doing along scientific lines than to display charts illustrating psychiatric problems, methods used, results obtained, and special equipment, arranged in an attractive manner as an exhibit.

DISTRIBUTION OF CASE HISTORIES

The case history method of teaching has become commonplace in medicine. Why not utilize this technique in our educational efforts? Selected case histories giving history, medical, psychiatric, and autopsy findings, and ending with a brief discussion could be mimeographed and distributed to the members of the district medical society monthly.

LETTERS TO PHYSICIANS

It is worth the time, trouble, and expense for any hospital to keep physicians fully informed about the patients they send in. A letter should be sent when the diagnosis is made. If the patient leaves the hospital the physician should be informed, and in case the patient dies, a copy of the autopsy protocol forwarded.

LIBRARY SERVICE

If the institution has a medical library, the services of the librarian may be offered to the profession. This is particularly valuable in rural communities. Outside physicians should be invited to visit the library and make use of its facilities.

CONSULTATION SERVICE

Many hospitals offer a consulting service to the outside physician. Psychiatrists are not available in rural communities. The hospital staff can render a real service to the general practitioner.

LABORATORY SERVICE

The hospital laboratory can be of inestimable benefit to the medical man who does not have such facilities at his command. Of course a charge should be made, but the value of the service is appreciated.

THE OPEN HOSPITAL

The mental patient is the only individual who cannot select his medical attendant. I see no reason why the mental hospital should not be open to any reputable practicing psychiatrist in the community. He should be able to follow his patient into the institution and carry out any treatment that he wishes. There is no justification for the custom that compels him to give up his patient at the door of the institution and turn him over to staff physicians. Such a policy would do much to allay the suspicion that exists in the minds of many relatives. If they could have their own physician in charge of the case it would give a sense of security that they do not have under present conditions.

Serving on the General Hospital Staff

The hospital psychiatrist who has a position on the staff of a general hospital is in a strategic position. He can do more to give the profession an understanding of what psychiatry means than is possible in any other way. His service may completely change the attitude of his fellow staff members.

Faculty Membership in Professional Schools

Schools of medicine, psychology, social work, and allied disciplines are turning more and more to the state hospital for psychiatric teaching. Fortunate is the mental institution which has a staff member on the faculty of a professional school. It enhances the dignity of the institution and places it in a position to make an educational contribution.

Social Service Agencies. *Courses for Social Workers*

This is a group of people who should receive special consideration from the mental hospital. Social workers need psychiatric instruction and the psychiatrist should be alert to make it possible for them to obtain it. Courses for social agencies will prove to be of great educational value, both to the worker and the institution. One of the principles underlying all educational measures is the fact that the community should bear some of the responsibility of adjusting patients in their homes. Social agencies should be encouraged to take over the supervision of discharged patients. As the institution extends itself into the community it will organize clinics, and such service to social workers will do a great deal to create a good hospital-society relationship.

Clergymen. The minister should know more about mental hygiene than he does. He has a real contribution to make in this field. He may and frequently does see the psychotic before anyone else. But if he is not sensitized to the problem of psychiatry, he may do incalculable damage. Psychiatric courses designed to assist the clergyman in his pastoral problems are helpful. The hospital has much to offer the church and the minister has something to give to psychiatry. One way to attract the interest of the community is to enlist the aid of church-women's organizations for services in visiting patients on the medical and surgical wards. Regular visiting will be of great benefit to the patient and will give those who carry it on an understanding of the hospital that they can get in no other way.

Nursing Organizations. It is important that the mental hospitals enlist the interest of this group in the problems of psychiatry. The earlier we begin an intensive educational program among nursing societies, the sooner we shall attract the proper type of nurse. Courses in psychiatry and psychiatric nursing, general hospital affiliation for undergraduates, and membership in these organizations by psychiatric nurses will be invaluable in opening up this nursing specialty.

Legal Associations. This profession needs psychiatric education. The lawyer should have sufficient understanding of the psychoses to protect himself against the psychotic who is constantly importuning him to redress imaginary wrongs. A closer relationship between psychiatric and legal societies would do much to clear up misunderstandings.

Police Departments. Here is a fruitful field for education. Many patients are brought to the institution by police officers and they are not always handled in the best way. In the larger cities police schools furnish an excellent opportunity for the hospital to get some educational propaganda to the department.

These and many other special community groups should be the object of educational efforts. An organized, systematic campaign of propaganda will bring rich rewards in the shape of increased confidence and better prestige in the community. This is mental hygiene.

Relatives and Friends of Patients. Every patient in a mental hospital has a circle of relatives and friends who may view the institution through the eye of suspicion that is so prevalent in the general community. Mental disease still places a stigma on those who are the victims of it, and the relatives of the patient participate in this fancied disgrace. Active and energetic efforts to break down this feeling will react directly for the benefit of the patient.

Letters to Relatives. The correspondence system of the hospital is a powerful factor in building morale among relatives. The hospital that keeps a relative informed as to the progress of the patient enjoys a better degree of confidence than the one which permits them to find out what they can. The following events should call for an informative letter:

When the Patient Is Received in the Hospital. This is a difficult time for the relatives of a patient. It is the time when they need understanding and sympathy. A letter of reassurance from the hospital will do a great deal to build confidence.

When the Patient Develops a Physical Illness. Any event in the life of the patient is worthy of a letter. This is proper from the standpoint of mental hygiene and as a protection for the hospital.

When He Recovers and Is Returned to His Ward. Relatives like good news as well as bad. When a patient has recovered from his illness it is good practice to inform them.

When a Patient Is Placed on the Danger List. Sudden deaths do not increase the confidence of the relatives in the hospital. Anticipating such occurrences is not only humanitarian but it is a factor in increasing the belief of the relatives in the medical skill of the staff.

When the Patient Is Taken Off the Danger List. The Danger List letter creates a situation of apprehension and dread. When the emergency has passed, the family should be notified.

Following the Death of a Patient. This is one of the most important letters a hospital can send. A note of personal sympathy at this time is always appreciated. Such a letter should contain information about the death, the rites of the church, disposition of clothing, and the result of the autopsy if there has been one.

When a Patient Escapes. Most hospitals notify relatives by telephone or telegraph. But a letter should confirm that notification, giving the full details and outlining what has been done to return him.

When He Returns from Escape. Many hospitals are rather lax in relieving the anxiety of relatives. The escape of a patient is always such a time.

When a Surgical Procedure Is Indicated. Naturally no surgery except emergency will be carried out without permission from the family. But such a letter should contain a detailed account of the condition which makes an operation necessary.

When the Operation Is Performed. Such a letter should be sent immediately after the operation. It is a time when everyone anticipates the worst. The hospital should relieve the worry.

When an Accident or Injury Occurs. Every accident, no matter how trivial, should be reported as soon as possible. Such a policy prevents some embarrassing situations. It is preferable for the hospital to inform the relative than to have the latter discover the injury first.

Letter of Advice When Patient Leaves the Hospital. When the patient leaves the hospital, a letter outlining the course of treatment for the patient should be sent. Such a letter indicates a spirit of coöperation on the part of the institution that cannot fail to impress a family. This letter should invite criticism as to the treatment the patient received while in the hospital and whether suggestions which will increase the efficiency of the hospital can be offered.

Booklets. The letter sent to the relative notifying him of the admission of the patient should have enclosed a booklet giving information about the hospital. This should deal with practical facts which will be of assistance to the relative in coöperating with the hospital. A booklet that would be particularly valuable to hand to relatives who bring patients is one which has detailed information about the admission procedure. It should be illustrated and go into complete detail of each step. Every hospital should have a plentiful supply of pamphlets giving information about mental disease.

Hospital Publication. There is no better educational medium for a mental hospital than a carefully edited paper sent to patients' relatives monthly. Such a publication should be attractively printed, and in addition to hospital news should have informative articles about mental disease and the management of the hospital. One of the best bulletins I have seen is a four-folder printed on a multigraph. It contained an article on the work of the pathological laboratory in relation to mental disease, a short story on accepting life, an occupational history of a patient, and a short biographical sketch of a staff member. It was written in readable newspaper style and well designed to create a good impression. The hospital mailed 1,500 of these papers each month to the relatives and friends of the patients. The mailing list was made up from the visiting records. This kind of paper is a valuable publicity medium for any institution.

Relatives' Meetings. A series of meetings of relatives and friends of patients always produces good will for the institution. These sessions are held at weekly intervals. On the particular visiting day that has been selected for the meeting, visitors coming in are handed an announcement giving the time and place of conference. Sufficient time should be allowed for visiting before the formal program. The subjects at these assemblies should deal with practical matters. The superintendent is the first speaker and he should bring home to his audience the practical difficulties of hospital administration, the necessity of complete coöperation on the part of relatives, the care of clothing, food supplies. If the hospital has a picture film or set of slides, they can be shown. Or the audience can be divided into small groups and shown points of interest in the hospital. Other meetings will deal with topics such as occupational therapy, psychotherapy, social service, psychiatric nursing, hydrotherapy, and food service. If this group is not too large they could be invited to have the evening meal with the patient and see what the food service is. Where hydrotherapy is being discussed, a pack demonstration could be given. There is so much misunderstanding about the use of the pack that an exhibition showing its correct application cannot fail to be impressive. A series of six such gatherings held once or twice each year will be a powerful factor in clearing up misunderstanding on the part of relatives and friends of patients.

Complaints of visitors frequently put the hospital personnel in an attitude of resentment. The psychiatrist, ward nurse, and superintendent are frequently on the defensive and appear guilty of something wrong because of their personal feeling towards the criticisms of visitors. Usually these are a manifestation of the emotional reaction of the visitors towards the fact that a relative has mental disease. The tragedy of illness may provoke an unreasonable revulsion that seizes on the hospital as a concrete human agency upon which they can precipitate their displeasure at life itself. An impersonal way of permitting visitors to make these complaints is to have accessible a question box into which comments and criticisms may be dropped. Much valuable information may be gained by the administrator in this manner. Records of complaints made to individuals should be accumulated. Social workers hear many of these comments and they should record each one for the general file. At intervals the superintendent goes through them and checks each one to ascertain that any inefficiencies leading to the complaint are adjusted.

Telephone Service. The telephone is an important link between hospital and community. The service is a good index of organization efficiency. Operators should be carefully selected for their pleasant manner, suitable voice, and particularly for the ability to maintain good poise under all sorts of trying conditions. They should certainly be thoroughly familiar with the departments of the hospital and its routine. They are preferably selected from the hospital personnel. The value of a telephone operator depends principally upon her capacity for keeping her temper and poise under all conditions. No set of rules can be formulated that will relieve her of the petty annoyances which occur at a hospital. These come from the peculiarities of human nature. A good operator will submit gracefully to such irritations.

Chapter 14

WHAT OF THE FUTURE?

WHAT can we see in the future of psychiatry in the light of the developments of the past? What will be the place of the hospital in this future evolution? Are the present policies of the mental hospital the best to insure a place in the future scheme of public health? These questions invariably arise in the mind of any administrator who has given the matter any thought. The question of whether he shall take an active or a passive rôle in attempting to guide the situation along definite lines is important. Should the mental hospital stand still and wait for the slow evolutionary process that will eventually change the entire picture, or would it be better to formulate a definite plan and work aggressively along specific lines?

One of the compensations for the labor involved in writing this book is the opportunity given the writer to indulge in phantasy about the future. It is my opinion that changes leading to a better understanding of the mental and emotional life of the individual will come about partly as a result of inevitable developments in our social and economic life and partly as a result of the attempts of psychiatrists to emphasize to the community the need for such understanding. In other words, what the mental hospital will be fifty years from now and the part psychiatry will play in world health affairs will be, to a considerable extent, dependent upon ourselves. The zeal with which administrators carry on crusades for proper principles, the pioneering spirit shown by the attempts to strike out into new and untried fields, and the courage shown in defending what we believe to be right will have a profound influence upon the future of psychiatry.

The state hospitals early assumed the leadership of American psychiatry. The history of the American Psychiatric Association would indicate that this statement is correct. The society was organized by hospital administrators and they represented the entire specialty in the community. As psychiatry developed more and more in the community, the hospital tried to maintain its traditional attitudes but without success. And finally, as a recognition of the broadening of psychiatric interest, the name of the association was changed from the American Association of Hospital Superintendents to American Medico-Psychological Association. Extramural psychiatrists with their new ideas of dynamic psychiatry and psychological medicine and therapy found themselves in the forefront of progress pointing the way, while some hospital administrators sat in their tents and sulked. Many of them refused to see the progressive changes that were coming about. The result of this attitude was that hospital psychiatry lagged far behind. The administrator withdrew more and more into his shell of isolation and the outsider ran faster and faster after many a will-o'-the-wisp which at first seemed to be substantial but many of which turned out to be fancies. Finally the reaction came, and the pendulum has swung back. The change of name of the association from American Medico-Psychological Association to American Psychiatric Association is a definite indication that psychiatry is turning back to the mental hospital, at least for support if not for leadership, and certainly to a recognition that the hospital has a place in the program.

With this trend and with our entire social life undergoing revision, the hospital is at the turning point in its history. It seems to me that the greatest obstacle to progress in psychiatry is the unwillingness of hospital administrators to build their organizations around the application of the available knowledge we possess. There seems to be a distinct rigidity of organization, a reluctance to move out of the even tenor of the way, and a tendency, in the enthusiasm for economy, to forget the patient who is being treated. Much of psychiatric progress will be in the hands of administrators because of their prestige with lay groups. The control of the situation is in their hands if they will exercise the power they possess. An emphasis upon the patient in community education will correct many existing evils and change the hospital from a segregating mechanism into an active agency for the treatment of mental disease. A broad outlook, a more active participation in social health movements, and scrutiny of present policies, with revision where needed, will again bring the mental hospital into a position of leadership.

Whether the practice of psychiatry is a science or an art or both will be determined in the future. At present it is largely an art, but with the extension of coördinated research it is possible that the scientific aspects of psychiatry will become dominant. Such a movement will bring together a group of eager, enthusiastic research workers representing all social sciences, working harmoniously together to discover the truth. Individual differences will disappear and mutual respect for each other will come when psychiatrists begin to apply their psychiatric knowledge to themselves as well as to the patient. I believe that coöperative research will be the plan to be followed in the future, with some agency acting as a clearing house for accumulated knowledge. Until psychiatry develops more of this spirit and eliminates some of the rugged individualism in research, we cannot hope to make rapid progress.

A program of this magnitude will be dependent, to a considerable extent, upon the administrator. If he is interested, sees in it a worth-while project, and will try to put it in operation, progress towards a solution of many problems will be more rapid. But if the policy of isolation continues, research will be retarded accordingly. This is a suitable time for state governments to take account of stock, overhaul the resources, and re-chart the course for the next hundred years. It is the responsibility of the administrator to change the thinking of the layman to the point where a more enlightened attitude and a better realization of the real issues involved will be the rule rather than the exception. When people understand that their relatives and friends must be cared for by experienced and well-trained individuals and that the encroachment of partisan politics into hospital administration takes its toll in a lessened chance for recovery of the patient, this practice will cease. But the responsibility of educating the community belongs to the administrator. I can visualize an enlightened state, free from the shackles of ignorance, superstition, and exploitation of the patient, bending its energies through well-trained organizations to increase the discharge rate and decrease the admission rate. If and when this is accomplished, we shall find that the criterion upon which each employee is judged will be on the basis of his contribution to the recovery of the patient.

There is a movement, which is slowly gaining impetus, to handle some of our psychiatric problems through special departments in general hospitals. A number of such departments have been organized in this country, and others will undoubtedly come into existence in the near future. The realization that physical disease has psychological concomitants is being more widely advertised than was the case in former years. In those general hospitals where psychiatric wards have been established the innovation has met with approval.

There is no reason why the general hospital should not bear its share of the burden of mental disease prevention. It is a problem of public health and as such is of interest to every agency interested in this important activity. This development is in line with the recent trend towards a more effective medical organization. American medical practice is highly individualistic but there is every reason to believe that through hospital and clinic a more widespread service will be rendered to the community at a lower cost. In 1929 approximately 15 per cent of the physicians in this country were a part of organized medicine and on a salary basis. The increase in the service rendered by general hospitals, the rapid development of industrial medical service, the growth of university health departments, and the organization of community health centers are all indications that the trend of medical practice is definitely towards less individualism and more organization. Governmental health activities have increased enormously during the past decade.

The uneven cost of medical care and distribution of medical service, the lack of care for chronic illnesses, and the inadequate emphasis on prevention are all forcing medical practice in the direction of organized medicine. The future will see some form of organization for medical practice. Psychiatry has already become a state function, and the growth of governmental participation in all health activity indicates the trend. All of these changes increase the activity and broaden the outlook of the general hospital. There is reason to believe that within the next two decades psychiatric departments in general hospitals will be the rule rather than the exception.

But, asks the thoughtful reader, will not this change the mental hospital from a receiving institution to a custodial hospital? It will if administrators permit it to happen. The service rendered will govern which institution the patient will turn to. If the mental hospital can give the best service the community will turn to it. If not, it will go to the general hospital.

But there is a field for both. The general hospital sees patients in the pre-psychotic stage. It has a unique opportunity to study the mental and emotional reactions to disease. There is evidence to show that these mechanisms during illness have an important influence upon the disease process. General hospitals have failed too long to accept their responsibilities in the field of psychiatry. They are in a favorable, strategic position to influence medical education and restore the art of medicine.

The era when the psychopathic hospital was thought to be the answer to all psychiatric problems is passing. While the ones that are now in existence are doing excellent work in research and training personnel, they have little effect upon the psychiatric problem as a whole. Most of these institutions have tended to become diagnostic clearing houses. The low bed capacity and high admission rate make it impossible for them to be anything else. The psychopathic hospital, as an independent unit, is a costly luxury and it is probable that the contribution it makes could be made more economically by some other agency, either the psychiatric department of the general hospital or a department of a mental hospital. To maintain a sorting center for patients with mental disease at an excessively high per capita cost is a doubtful procedure.

If a mass movement against mental disorder is to come, all professional groups dealing with human beings will have to participate in it. In my opinion the mental hygiene of the future will not be carried on by special groups of psychiatrists. True, training facilities will always have to be maintained, but the actual contact with patients in the early stages of maladjustment will be through the general practitioner, teacher, juvenile court judge, probation officer, police officer, social worker, clergyman, Y.M.C.A., Y.W.C.A., Boy and Girl Scout leaders, Boy and Girl Club leaders, and parents. Each of these groups has a direct responsibility in the field of mental hygiene.

The physician who carries on medical practice in the community will have had a better education in mental hygiene and psychiatry than those of past generations. Already there is apparent a swing away from the extreme scientific attitude in medicine. Leaders recognize that the rapid growth of cults and irregular methods of healing represents a community need for help that the profession has not been able to furnish. Restrictive legislation will never stop the onward march of these cults. It is the physicians themselves who must recognize that the individual is not a machine which can be reduced to a mathematical formula but an unpredictable, unstable, and irrational mass of protoplasm, and that the emotions of men rule their behavior, cause many illnesses, and generally bring discord into their social and personal lives. Medical schools must become cognizant of their responsibility in the field of social medicine. Merely creating a department of psychiatry in the medical school will not bring results. I am not sure that any changes need be made. But what must come is a demand on the part of the school that every faculty member who teaches students know and appreciate the significance of mental mechanisms in disease processes and stress their importance to the students. In other words, the medical teacher must know more about social medicine and the art of applying his scientific knowledge than he does today. When this attitude arrives in the medical school psychiatry will be a respectable specialty and the mass action on mental disease will have begun.

Philanthropic organizations will be more generous in their subsidy of teaching and research in mental disease. There is a definite trend in this direction even now. But the tendency is to give financial aid to existing organizations rather than to inaugurate new projects.

Education will understand the obligation it has to teach children to live instead of merely acquiring a mass of factual knowledge. The teacher will look below the surface indications for her explanation of the unusual conduct of the child.

She will begin to see the latter, not as a mere receptacle for the forcible implantation of so much geography, arithmetic, and grammar, but as a human organism filled with deep and powerful instincts, drives, hopes, and ambitions. The educational process will be used as a tool for increasing the happiness of life rather than for the mere acquisition of knowledge as an end in itself. School systems will recognize the importance of the first eight years of the child's life and will place the best teacher in charge of the first grade. Promotion will be from the high school down into the grades, and the highest paid teacher will be the one who has the child during his first year in school. Finally, the selection of those who are to train our children will be on the basis of training, experience, and fitness for the job rather than on the basis of political affiliation, as is frequently the case now. The teacher will have a social status that is commensurate with her importance in our social scheme.

The field of juvenile delinquency is so wrapped up in our social structure that it becomes increasingly difficult to separate out the rôle of any one particular agency. But the juvenile court certainly has a vital responsibility in the mental hygiene of the future. If these courts are actually to make any impression upon crime in a preventive way, men must be trained to handle the problems that come before them from the standpoint of the child specialist rather than from the point of view of the law. A mere legal training will not be sufficient for the juvenile court judge of the future. He will have a conception and understanding of the social implications of crime and will understand the psychological reactions on the part of the child to these situations. Less of the police and legal attitude and more understanding of the individual will characterize the future juvenile court judge. And the court will not be an adjunct to a police court but will be a full-time job for specially trained judges and probation officers.

The church has a responsibility in the field of mental hygiene which it has consistently overlooked for ages. But the whole field of ministerial education will have to be revised before the clergyman is prepared to carry out that responsibility. Emphasis upon technical theology will give way to the consideration and understanding of those subtle and mysterious forces within the individual which regulate human behavior. The clergyman of the future will have had clinical training during his educational period, and this experience will enable him to serve his parishioners on a basis of understanding rather than a theological formula. He will be a factor, as a minister, in mental hygiene.

The future social worker, with a background of psychological and psychiatric training, will be able to handle those problems which confront her with an appreciation of the mental mechanisms involved. She will look upon the mental hospital as a constructive agency which can help her to solve these problems, not by locking up all the people about her but by a coöperative effort to assist in their adjustment in the community.

All of these groups, under the leadership of the hospital, will be the mental hygienists of the future. They will be psychiatrically minded and make up that mass movement against mental disorder which I believe to be essential before any real achievement can come.

Extramural child and adult psychiatric clinics will develop under the auspices of the state government, supported jointly by the state and town. That movement is represented by activities in New Jersey. I believe it is quite possible that the various states may be split into districts much as the Public Health officials work, and that traveling clinics may be organized. Rural districts are particularly in need of trained psychiatric personnel.

The parent of tomorrow will be a more enlightened individual and better able to handle the problems of childhood than he is today. The complete swing away from discipline towards a complete freedom for the child will turn back to a more common-sense attitude in which the necessity for inculcating in the child a respect for law and order is recognized but a proper degree of self-expression is permitted.

There is no gain to be made through wholesale sterilization procedures, but future legislation will recognize the necessity of such measures in individual cases. The present sentimental attitude towards such plans will, it is to be hoped, give way to a scientific scrutiny of the facts, both biological and psychological.

I see the state mental hospital of the future as a powerful and leading factor in the public health of the community, its interests broad and far-reaching and its leadership unquestioned by those whom it serves. It will control the community clinics which I believe will be dotted all over the country, it will represent the finest type of medical service, and it will be the coördinating agency which ties up all activities dealing with human beings. The hospital will have the complete confidence and respect of society and it will be free from the domination of partisan politics and the manipulation of its work by unscrupulous politicians. Psychiatric administration will represent a career for which men train rigorously. The opportunity is here for making the initial step towards this goal. And what the mental hospital of tomorrow is depends very largely upon the administrator of today, his hopes, fears, ideals, purposes, and drives. His organizing ability can be made infinitely more productive if he believes that administrative psychiatry consists of a great deal more than "bossing" people.

BIBLIOGRAPHY

1. Herzog, Rudolph. "Die Wunderheilungen von Epidauros." *Philologus,* Supplementband, *22,* No. 3, 1931.
2. Regis, E. *A Practical Manual of Mental Medicine.* Translated by H. M. Bannister. 2nd Ed. Utica, New York, 1894.
3. O'Donoghue, Edward Geoffrey. *The Story of Bethlehem Hospital from Its Foundation in 1247.* E. P. Dutton, New York, 1915.
4. Tuke, Samuel. *Description of the Retreat,* York, 1813. P. 175.
5. Anonymous. "Moral Treatment of Insanity." *American Journal of Insanity, 4:* 1, 1847.
6. Quoted in "Moral Treatment of Insanity." *American Journal of Insanity, 4:* 7, 1847.
7. Tiffany, Francis. *Life of Dorothea Lynde Dix.* Houghton, Mifflin & Company, Boston, 1896. P. 54.
8. Pratt, George K. "Twenty Years of the National Committee for Mental Hygiene." *Mental Hygiene, 14:* 399, 1930.
9. Ruggles, Arthur H. "Twenty-five Years of Work." *Mental Hygiene, 19:* 1, 1935.
10. *J.A.M.A. 104:* 1081, 1935.
11. Treadway, W. L. "Federal Activities in Care of the Mentally Ill." *Proc. Annual Congress of Medical Education,* A.M.A., Chicago, 1931. Pp. 3-8.
12. Hamilton, Samuel W. "State Institutions and Their Relation to Medicine in General." *Ibid.* Pp. 8-10.
13. Peterson, Frederick, Haines, Walter S., and Webster, Ralph W. *Legal Medicine and Toxicology.* W. B. Saunders, Philadelphia, 1923. Vol. I. 2nd Ed.
14. Emerson, Harrington. *The Twelve Principles of Efficiency.* The Engineering Magazine Company, New York, 1919. 5th Ed. Pp. 31 seq.
15. Holmes, Oliver Wendell. Quoted by Clendening, Logan, *Behind the Doctor.* Garden City Publishing Company, Garden City, New York, 1933. Foreword.

16. Tead, Ordway. *Human Nature and Management*. McGraw-Hill Book Company, New York, 1929. P. 149.
17. Gilbreth, F. B. Quoted by Shefferman, Nathan W. *Employment Methods*. Ronald Press Company, New York, 1920. P. 228.
18. Hoskins, R. G. "Dementia Praecox—A Simplified Formulation." *J.A.M.A., 96:* 1209, 1931.
19. Davis, John E. "The Attendant in Mental Re-education." *Mental Hygiene, 18:* 629, 1934.
20. White, William A. *The Principles of Mental Hygiene*. Macmillan, New York, 1919. P. 75.
21. Committee on The Grading of Nursing Schools. *Nursing Schools Today and Tomorrow*. New York, 1934. P. 45.
22. Simon, H. "Active Treatment of Patients in Insane Asylums." *Allg. Ztschr. f. Psychiat. 87:* 97, 1927, and *ibid. 90:* 69 and 245, 1929.
23. Kellogg, J. H. *Rational Hydrotherapy*. Modern Medicine Publishing Company, Battle Creek, Michigan, 1923. 17th Ed.
24. McDougall, William. *Outline of Abnormal Psychology*. Charles Scribner, New York, 1926. P. 117.
25. Dembo, T. and Hanfmann, E. "The Value of an Orientation Letter for Newly Admitted Patients." *Psychiat. Quarterly, 8:* 703, 1934.
26. *Annual Report of the Committee on Mental Hospitals*, American Association of Psychiatric Social Workers, 1932-1934. Pp. 7-17.
27. Taft, Jessie. "Qualifications of the Social Worker." *Mental Hygiene, 3:* 426, 1919.
28. 72nd Report of the Friends' Retreat, York, 1866. Quoted in *American Journal of Insanity, 25:* 502, 1869.
29. Whitehead, A. N. *The Aims of Education and Other Essays*. Macmillan, New York, 1929. P. 6.
30. Stewart, Isabel M. "How Shall We Plan the Program of Study?" *American Journal of Nursing, 35:* 575, 1935.
31. Kilpatrick, William Heard. "The Educational Challenge." *American Journal of Nursing, 35:* 613, 1935.
32. Leonard, Marion. "Committee on Clinical Instruction of the National League of Nursing Education." *American Journal of Nursing, 35:* 688, 1935.

33. *Ward Manual for Employees.* Worcester State Hospital, Care and Handling of Patients. P. 1. (Mimeographed.)

34. Alexander, George H. "Sedatives: Types, Uses, and Dangers." *American Journal of Nursing, 35:* 222, 1935.

35. Thielbar, Frances C. "Sedatives and Nursing Care." *Ibid.* P. 229.

36. Somerville, John. "The Forgotten Problem: Aims in Science." *Philosophy of Science, 2:* 246, 1935.

37. Keeler, Ralph Welles. "The Significance and Function of Publicity for Hospitals." *Modern Hospital, 20:* 429, 1923.

INDEX